you can heal yourself

Trusted Advice for a Healthier Life
from Harvard Medical School

you can

heal

yourself

A Guide to Physical and
Emotional Recovery After
Injury or Illness

Julie Silver, MD

 St. Martin's Griffin ⚓ New York

www.stmartins.com

The information in this book is not intended to replace the advice of the reader's own physician or other medical professional. You should consult a medical professional in matters relating to health, especially if you have existing medical conditions, and before starting, stopping, or changing the dose of any medication you are taking. Individual readers are solely responsible for their own health care decisions. The author and the publisher do not accept responsibility for any adverse effects individuals may claim to experience, whether directly or indirectly, from the information contained in this book.

The fact that an organization or Web site is mentioned in the book as a potential source of information does not mean that the author or the publisher endorse any of the information they may provide or recommendations they may make.

The stories in this book are composite, fictional accounts based on the experiences of many individuals. Similarities to any real person or persons are coincidental and unintentional.

Library of Congress Cataloging-in-Publication Data

Silver, J. K. (Julie K.), 1965–
    You can heal yourself : a guide to physical and emotional recovery after injury or illness / Julie K. Silver.
        p. cm.
    ISBN 978-0-312-60580-3 (pbk.)
    1. Medical rehabilitation—Popular works.   2. Medicine, Physical—Popular works.   3. Healing—Popular works.   I. Title.
    RM930.S553 2012
    617.03—dc23   2011035938

First Edition: February 2012

10 9 8 7 6 5 4 3 2 1

To everyone who needs to heal

contents

acknowledgments

I am grateful to my publishing and medical colleagues who have offered me their advice and wisdom. I thank my doctors, nurses, and other healthcare providers for their expertise and empathy. Love and gratitude to my family and friends for nurturing me in sickness and in health.

Focus on You

chapter 1

Listen to Your Healing Voice

Kathleen sat in the cold metal chair of the hospital waiting room anxiously watching the organized chaos. The room itself was unattractive, with graying tile floors and not enough seats, which is why she was sitting on a folding chair. Finally, the nurse called her name, loud enough for everyone to hear, though the others seemed oblivious. Kathleen jumped up, eager to move away from the crowded room. The nurse led her to a tiny changing room where she hung her clothes and donned a hospital gown. The next stop was a private room where an ultrasound technician was waiting.

The technician was efficient in her routine but then she hesitated over a suspicious area. "I'll be right back," she said. Kathleen waited. Finally, the technician came back. "The doctor will be here in a minute. I just want him to check something." When the doctor arrived, he stood across the room as the technician moved the ultrasound machine over Kathleen's body. "This is what I wanted to show you," she told him. "That's nothing, just a lymph node," he explained curtly and then left the room without ever speaking to Kathleen.

Kathleen dressed silently, relieved to be going home. Relieved that everything was fine. Or at least, she told herself that she was relieved. But, the truth was, she didn't feel relieved. She was worried. Yes, the waiting room *was* ugly and unfriendly. The nurse *was* indifferent to the rules regarding patient privacy; the doctor *was* arrogant and rude. Still, did that mean that she couldn't trust the test and the doctor's conclusion?

Over the next couple of weeks, Kathleen decided that she didn't trust the doctor. He obviously hadn't cared and she wanted to at least find a doctor who seemed to care. One she could trust to help her if something was wrong. So, she made an appointment to see another doctor, a woman in a different hospital who came highly recommended.

The woman was a breast surgeon, and she was used to looking at all kinds of lumps and bumps from worried women. This time, the waiting room was more welcoming, the nurse more discreet, and the doctor more caring. Kathleen had the tests repeated. The doctor told her, "I can't feel anything when I examine you, and the tests are all negative. There is no evidence that anything is wrong."

Kathleen left, and again was relieved. Relieved to be going home to her baby and other children. Relieved to tell her husband that all was well. Relieved that she had found a doctor who didn't stand across the room and dismiss her concerns with barely a nod in her direction. And so, she went back to her regular life. With three children to raise, there wasn't much time to worry. Besides, she was fine. Two doctors had told her so. Multiple tests had been normal. She was fine. Or was she?

Two years later, Kathleen realized that she was still worried. She had been worried off and on, but for the most part had convinced herself that she must be acting a bit hypochondriacally. After all, she was young and healthy. Too young for a serious health problem—even the tests confirmed this.

She went back to the female breast surgeon. More tests ensued. This time, her doctor said, "You were right. You have cancer."

Kathleen is my middle name, and this is my story.

Entering the Healing Zone

Many people have asked me, "How did you know something was wrong when your doctors and the tests didn't show anything?" The simple answer is that we all have incredible knowledge about our own bodies that far exceeds what anyone else could ever know. This doesn't mean that doctors and medical tests aren't extremely valuable. They are. But, they don't always know or reveal what you know about your body. You have amazing and very intimate knowledge about your body, which makes you a powerful healer when it comes to healing yourself. Of course, it would be wonderful if you weren't in need of healing, but all of us enter what the late author Susan Sontag called the "kingdom of the sick" at various points in our lives. In a vivid description in *Illness as Metaphor*, Sontag wrote:

> Illness is the night-side of life, a more onerous citizenship. Everyone who is born holds dual citizenship, in the kingdom of the well and in the kingdom of the sick. Although we all prefer to use only the good passport, sooner or later each of us is obliged, at least for a spell, to identify ourselves as citizens of that other place.

The great irony with cancer is that usually you begin treatment feeling great but know that something terrible is going on inside your body. By the end of treatment you are physically debilitated but often feel grateful that treatment was even possible. In *Flying Crooked,* Jan Michael describes it this way: "Such a weird disease, creeping through your body without your noticing. First you have lumps, but you feel fine. You're whisked into hospital and they mutilate you, and suddenly, you're not fine at all."

As a cancer patient, I had to live in what I call "the Healing Zone" for a couple of years. The Healing Zone is a place where a lot of patients get stuck and many never heal optimally—instead, accepting a "new normal" and a higher-than-needed level of pain, fatigue, weakness, disability, and emotional turmoil.

As a physician who specializes in rehabilitation medicine, I have worked for many years with patients who are in the Healing Zone. I treat people with many different kinds of conditions, including—but not limited to—cancer, stroke, multiple sclerosis, traumatic brain injuries, sports injuries, neck and low back pain, and just about any other condition in which healing is required. I also treat individuals with orthopedic conditions that range from sprained ankles and knees to serious multitrauma injuries due to car accidents and physical violence.

As a cancer patient, when I had been given my last chemotherapy treatment, my oncologist told me, "Now get on with the rest of your life." This was simultaneously both heartening and disheartening. I was delighted to move forward, but I was a physical wreck. Emotionally, I was depleted. My doctor's work was done—he had rid me of my cancer and, save for the occasional checkup to be sure it did not reappear, I was on my own. I pause here to say that I had outstanding care and that my doctors were dedicated and smart, and worked hard to save my life. However, like so many people, there came a time when I was on my own and still in need of healing.

Many patients turn to self-help books during times of illness, and I was no different. During my recovery, I searched for books that focused on healing—both physically and emotionally. I was surprised to find that despite the hundreds of books on cancer, there wasn't a single book devoted to how survivors could best heal. Because I wanted a guide, and I knew that there were many others who could benefit, too, I wrote *After Cancer Treatment: Heal Faster, Better, Stronger*—a book specifically for cancer survivors about how to heal optimally. As I wrote it, however, I realized that much of the advice was the same as what I was giving to my patients who had many different illnesses and injuries. This is because there are many universal healing principles that really work to help us optimally recover both physically and emotionally.

Helping people to heal optimally is what physiatrists do every day. Physiatrists (doctors who specialize in "rehabilitation medicine"—technically referred to as Physical Medicine and Rehabilitation, or PM&R) focus on how to bridge the gap between what one's body can do to heal without any assistance and what one's body can do with evidence-based medical advice that allows for *optimal* healing.

My story is similar to many people's stories, regardless of whether they were diagnosed with cancer or some other illness. There is so much untapped potential for healing and far too many of us struggle with weakness, fatigue, pain, and other symptoms that can be improved or sometimes eliminated altogether. There is no doubt that any kind of illness or injury negatively impacts our lives. As you read this book, remember that illness makes you feel vulnerable and healing makes you powerful.

Beginning to Heal

Physiatrists tend to have a very "holistic" approach to healing and recognize the importance of using many different treatment strategies as well as an individual's inner resources. So, as I began to heal, I thought about my years of medical training and practice. Faced with my desire to recover quickly and to feel physically and emotionally stronger, I had to distill an incredible amount of knowledge into some basic healing principles that I could follow. I was too ill to think about, much less implement, all of the various healing methods I knew. Instead, I had to decide what are the *best* ways? What are the main principles in healing, and how can I achieve them with the least effort?

In order to figure this out, I had to start really listening to my healing voice. This is something I tell my patients all the time: Listen to your body; what is it telling you? Try thinking about these questions (write down the answers if you want to):

1. Are you in pain?
2. Where does it hurt?
3. When does it hurt?
4. What makes it better?
5. What makes it worse?
6. Do you feel fatigued?
7. Do you have any problems falling asleep, staying asleep, or sleeping well?
8. When are you most fatigued?
9. When are you least fatigued?
10. What makes you less tired?
11. What makes you more tired?
12. Other than sleep, are there things you can do to pick up your energy?
13. Do you feel weak?
14. What is the weakest part of your body?

15.   What is the strongest part of your body?
16.   What parts of your body do you have confidence in and trust to work well?
17.   What parts of your body are you worried about?
18.   What makes you currently feel sad? Worried? Anxious? Depressed? Angry?
19.   What makes you currently feel happy? Relieved? Peaceful?
20.   What do you think will help you to heal as well as possible?

When I start asking a patient who has come to my office in pain these types of questions, it's not uncommon that he or she has to stop and think about the answers. When we're busy living our lives, we often don't really pay attention to how we feel physically and emotionally. Perhaps it seems a little narcissistic—overly focused on one's self. Or, maybe we're just too busy. Possibly, it's just easier to think about other things. Whatever the reason, in order to begin to heal, listening to your healing voice is an important first step. You know your body better than anyone else. You have intimate knowledge of how your body works and feels that no doctor could ever have, no matter how many years of medical training she had.

While this book is on how to heal yourself, and I acknowledge that you know more about your body than any physician ever could, it still is really important to get good medical advice. As a patient, I relied on my physicians to help me. Their care was essential to my well-being, and while I think individuals can do a great deal to help themselves heal, I also believe in getting excellent medical advice all along the way.

Before I could write *After Cancer Treatment: Heal Faster, Better, Stronger,* I had to work on healing myself. This process forced me to synthesize the medical research and develop a recovery plan for cancer survivors. When I felt well enough and began to write the book, I thought about how the healing principles are really the same for the vast majority of people I treat. There are core principles that I used to heal myself, described in that book, and discuss daily with patients who come to my office. These core principles are based on thousands of research studies and many years of my listening to patients tell me what helps them and what doesn't.

You Can Heal Yourself is based on the best medical research currently available along with common sense, intuition, and a lot of experience treating people who are in need of physical and emotional healing. In conventional medicine, what we refer to as "evidence-based" medicine, research is paramount. We rely heavily on the results of studies that show us what works and what doesn't. However, there are many gaps in research, and to fill these voids doctors utilize common sense, intuition, and experience. These skills are what make up the "art" of medicine. A skilled physician is both a scientist and an artist.

Before this book came out, I put the cover of it in a slide presentation I was giving to a group of cancer survivors. Afterward, the director of the cancer center asked me whether this book was about curing cancer, even at the end stage. She cornered me with obvious criticism in her voice. After all, is it really fair to encourage people to heal if they don't have a good prognosis? I explained to her I don't want to suggest that every illness has a cure, but that too many people suffer far more than they need to—whether they currently live with an illness or are simply suffering from the after-effects of one.

She brought up late stage cancer (stage 4), which I think is a worthwhile example to explore. Certainly, some people who are diagnosed with stage 4 cancer will be cured. Lance Armstrong is an example of someone who was cured de-spite the cancer spreading to distant parts of his body (that's the criteria for stage 4—distant spread of the cancer, or *me-tastasis*). However, many people with stage 4 cancer will not be cured, but rather will live with cancer as a chronic condi-tion. Prostate cancer is typically diagnosed in men over the age of fifty years. Often it is diagnosed in the early stages, but sometimes the cancer has spread. It is not uncommon for men with prostate cancer that is stage 4 to suffer from debilitating side effects of treatment but still have a relatively good prog-nosis. This means they can benefit from healing but may live for years with cancer as a chronic condition.

Statistics don't always predict any one person's outcome. Statistics give us information about what may happen, but there are no guarantees. Putting a positive spin on this means it's important to remember that even when the prognosis is grim, there are outliers—people who don't follow the statis-tics. It's usually not clear why this happens, but giving every person the opportunity to live as healthy a life as possible is critical. It's difficult to predict how or why some people "beat the odds." For example, in 1988, Katherine Russell Rich was diagnosed with breast cancer. Five years later, she was told by her doctors that her cancer had progressed to stage 4, and she had less than two years to live. For many years, she has taught at a publishing course that I direct at Harvard Medical School. Though she clearly has had some health issues, Kathy travels from New York to Boston and teaches memoir writing—which gets rave reviews from the attendees.

In 2010, Kathy wrote an article for *The New York Times* titled "17 Years Later, Stage 4 Survivor Is Savoring a Life Well Lived." I can't explain Kathy's longevity, but what is important to note is that it's not always easy to predict what will happen with people when they are ill. Even if they live with a very serious illness, during their lifetime they deserve to live with the highest possible level of health. Every day that they can feel stronger and have more energy and less fatigue is worthwhile. Year after year, Kathy has had the physical and emotional strength to travel and teach. She has been a powerful influence on the lives of many people.

So, although I understand the cancer center director's concerns, I want to share with readers that healing is not always about curing an illness, but rather is focused on living the best life you can despite certain health circumstances that may be out of your control.

* * *

In this book, I combine the art and science of medicine into strategies that will allow you to heal yourself as well as possible—physically and emotionally—no matter what problems you are facing. I don't focus on "cure," but rather on helping your mind and your body to be as strong as possible, even if you live with a medical condition such as cancer, diabetes, or arthritis. This information will help you tap into and mobilize your own healing resources. These resources will assist you in "bumping up" your level of health and becoming a little, or hopefully even a lot, stronger, even if there isn't a cure for whatever it is that you are suffering with. And, the first step is simply to listen to your healing voice: What is it telling you?

Healing Strategies

Analyze Your Weaknesses and Study Your Strengths

As you begin to listen to your healing voice, it's important to focus not only on the negative messages that you are receiving, but also the positive ones. What problems are you having and what is working well for you? Try this exercise to help you focus on where you might have room to heal and at the same time appreciate your mind and your body right now.

1. List three ways that you wish your body would function better.

2. List three ways that you wish your mind (or emotions) would function better.
3. List three things that you like about your body and trust it to do well.
4. List three things that you like about your mind (or emotions) and trust it to do well.

chapter 2

Begin to Heal

One day an elderly man lost control of his car near where I used to work. The car careened out of control in the parking lot and smashed through a storefront window. A young woman who had just started college never saw the car coming. She heard the breaking glass and then everything went black. She woke up with family surrounding her hospital bed and was relieved to see her mother smiling down at her. But something was missing: her leg.

Despite a normal period of tremendous grief and many hours spent in physical therapy, she carried on with her plans to attend college. There is a beauty and a grace about her that is truly indescribable. People are drawn to her warmth and her character. In short, she has the grace of someone who has healed as well as she can and has now gone on with her life. She is not a tragic heroine but an accomplished woman who has successfully navigated serious adversity.

For years, before I had to face my own healing challenges, I would marvel at my patients—particularly those who approached healing with what I can only define as "grace." Through my observations, I found that the grace with which people dealt with illness had little to do with their diagnosis, whether they were male or female, how old they were, or any other objective factors. This young woman and many others like her were role models for me as I faced cancer and the toxic treatments I needed to save my life.

Healing is a process that you can "own" but not completely control. There is always the opportunity to heal optimally but not necessarily completely. While embracing strategies to improve your health is important for your healing journey, there is no doubt that you will likely feel more or less discouraged at various times during this process. Of course, there are times that you may focus on what you can't change and wonder, "Why is this happening?" You may be angry, depressed, frustrated, or have a combination of many other emotions. This is all normal and the goal here is simply to do the best that you can to accept what you can't change and focus your attention on how you can help yourself heal.

You may be thinking, how can I accept what has happened to me? We all want to be whole and happy. Claudia Osborn is a doctor who was hit by a car while cycling. She sustained a traumatic brain injury and wrote about her incomplete recovery. In her memoir, *Over My Head*, she describes how she wanted to again be "the real me." Claudia writes:

> One word, hiding in my unconscious, lying in wait on the periphery of my knowledge, had stripped me of hope and shattered my dreams. Permanent. How could

I continue to live with this deficient brain, continue to exist in the unrecognizable, undesirable being? My head injury was bearable only because it was temporary. Permanent injury meant I had already lost. My job. My identity. My life. I was not this damaged shell of a person. I couldn't be. I remembered and loved the person I was. That was the real me.

It is normal to grieve over what you have lost and to be worried about what the future holds for you and your family. I encourage my patients to grieve; however, I also tell them that they can turn their worry into an advantage. Perhaps this is the reason you are reading this book. Maybe being a bit worried helps you to remember to take your medicine every day. Despite feeling worried, you can shape your attitude into one that will help you heal. Nazi death camp survivor, Viktor Frankl, reminded us, "Everything can be taken away from a man but one thing: the last of the human freedoms—to choose one's attitude in any given set of circumstances."

Worry is closely aligned with uncertainty, and uncertainty is practically synonymous with illness. No one with a health issue is free from the worry associated with uncertainty. While it is true that much of what we count on day to day is actually uncertain, illness takes this unpredictability to a higher level and doesn't allow for even the illusion of knowing what the future holds.

But uncertainty, and the worry associated with it, doesn't have to rule your life. No one has the recipe for how to live a certain life. We can make plans and many of those will be realized, but not all. Instead, the antidote to uncertainty is to minimize how much you let it haunt you in your daily routine. It is possible to laugh and to seek enjoyment and fulfillment, despite difficult circumstances. I don't want to minimize people's genuine suffering but rather to point out that pain and suffering are often constant companions, but they can be accompanied by contentment, peace, and even joy. No matter what you need to heal from, the principles of survivorship are remarkably similar across the continuum. After surviving a serious illness or injury, the next step is to face reality and decide how you are going to live. Ideally, this will include using some strategies that will help you to heal.

Don't Underestimate Your Ability to Heal

Though healing may take a long time and might not be complete, it is easy to underestimate what you'll be able to accomplish in your quest for better health (even your doctors may underestimate your potential). For example, in August 2001, my uncle, who was then the Olympic sports editor for *USA Today,* called me at home and asked if I would be willing to review the X-rays of then the most recognizable alpine skier in the world, two-time Olympic and world champion, Hermann Maier, who had been thrown from his motorcycle into a ditch when he collided with a car in front of him. Maier was airlifted to a hospital in Salzburg, where surgeons spent seven hours trying to save his right leg. Following the surgery, his kidneys were failing and there was still the possibility he would have to have his leg amputated.

After hearing about the accident, in which "The Herminator" sustained nerve damage in both of his legs, and looking at the X-rays of his right leg fractures (both bones in the lower leg were crushed), I thought that this was likely a career-ending injury for this legend. I gave a quote for the article: "The major concern is infection and will be for quite a while." I also mentioned that while the bones would heal fairly quickly, other more disabling injuries might be problematic (for example, he might have permanent nerve damage to his legs). After doing this interview, I didn't think much more about Maier until a short four months later when I read that he was back on skis. At that time he had to wear a special boot to protect his right shin, where skin from his left upper arm was grafted. Then, to my amazement, just seventeen months after this truly horrific accident, Maier won a World Cup Super-G in Kitzbuhel, Austria.

Few people would have predicted Maier's amazing recovery, yet his story is not entirely unique. Cyclist Lance Armstrong's story may have made international news when he won the Tour de France after a difficult physical recovery from advanced testicular cancer that had spread to his brain, but there are many other stories of unsung heroes or "regular Joes and Janes" who have worked to heal themselves as well as possible.

Your ability to weather setbacks has a lot to do with your perspective. Although most people envision healing as steps they take to improve their health without ever having a setback, the truth is that this is rarely the way it happens. There are often unwanted stops or detours along the way. Your recovery might feel like a "two steps forward and one step back" process or perhaps a two steps forward and then a halt to the progression with no further forward or backward motion for a while. Just knowing that you will almost certainly experience healing plateaus or setbacks can go a long way to helping you prepare for and overcome them. Because this is such a common pattern, I will spend more time later in this book discussing how to handle healing plateaus and setbacks.

Take Back Control

Before we move on to the healing strategies, it's important to acknowledge that any change in our health status throws us into a state of turmoil and can make us feel out of control. A new diagnosis makes us feel vulnerable and distrust our bodies. The road from vulnerability to empowerment is not always easy. However, the purpose of this book is to help you take back some control—step by step. Working toward physical and emotional recovery is an important goal that can help take you from powerlessness to empowerment.

While this book is designed to give you the information you need to heal well, it is also important to realize that you don't have to do everything perfectly (such as, eat an ideal diet all the time, adhere to a strict exercise regimen, never miss a workout, and so on). In the past, I have described this as a rule I made up called the Bill Clinton "one wrong move" rule. Perhaps you recall the incident in 1997 when then president Clinton arrived at Hobe Sound, Florida, and was looking forward to a golf excursion later in the day. While attempting to go to his guest cottage, he descended a flight of stairs and his heel caught on a step. He stumbled, and as he fell his leg made a loud snapping noise that others reported hearing. Clinton ended up with a torn tendon that required surgery.

Quite literally, Clinton took one wrong step. While one wrong step can certainly cause an injury, in the recovery phase, there is no one wrong step. It simply doesn't apply— which means that you won't be able to do (or not do) one thing and have a major problem. If you don't exercise regularly, you have a period of depression, you like to eat dessert, or you decide that you don't want to tap into the Universe (or spiritual) reservoirs, you will still be able to heal. So, don't be concerned if you don't follow all the strategies in this book. Rather, think of them as steps to healing as well as you possibly can. An ancient proverb declares, "If fate throws a knife at you, there are two ways of catching it—by the blade or by the handle." Embracing strategies that help you to mend as well as possible is a way of catching fate's knife by the handle.

Adopting some healing strategies is forward movement in your journey. It is also part of transitioning from critical illness to better health. Yet, there is no doubt that transitions are filled with uncertainty and they make us uncomfortable.

They can make us feel worried and wary. Unfortunately, there is no getting around it—if you are in need of healing, this is a period of transition. During this time, some people become immobilized due to fear and uncertainty. Others will take that negative energy and use it to help them recover.

For everyone who faces a serious medical condition, the road to healing is filled with choices, and a commitment to spend the time on recovery is an important one to make. As you read this book and work toward healing, there will be "crossroads"—different paths you can take. There isn't necessarily one right path and all the rest are wrong. Rather, there are simply multiple ways that you can approach your recovery based on a variety of factors including your medical condition and your personal philosophies and character. Keep in mind that while I will encourage you to adopt some healing strategies, the Bill Clinton "one wrong move" rule does not apply. Which means that you don't have to do things perfectly to heal well.

Plan Your Work and Work Your Plan

Setting goals is really helpful when it comes to healing. If you don't define what you want to achieve, then it's difficult to accomplish any given task. Goals offer you a way to measure where you are now, and a vision of what you want to achieve in the future. Or, as the famous baseball coach Yogi

Berra once said, "If you don't know where you are going, you might wind up someplace else."

Goals provide structure and purpose. A healing journey without goals is akin to driving on an unpaved road, whereas goals lead you down a paved path. You can heal without goals, but it's far easier to accomplish something if you know what it is you want to achieve.

When I give speeches, I often ask the audience to participate by listing their three most important health goals— physical and/or emotional. I encourage them to write down goals that they have some control over. Then, I ask them what they did last week to work toward accomplishing their most important goals. Not surprisingly, many people start to laugh and realize that they haven't done anything to work toward what they consider extremely important. This is followed by my asking them to write down what they can do this week to work toward what they've identified as their most important goals. Most people participate enthusiastically and realize that today is a new day, and there is an opportunity to focus on the things that matter most to them.

Reading this book can provide a new beginning to your healing journey. Congratulations on a good start. As you read each chapter and the different healing strategies, keep up the momentum by setting some goals. There is no better time to start than today. In creating goals for yourself, consider the strategies in this book. Which ones do you think will help you? Trust your own instincts.

Because recovery is not entirely predictable, goals should be flexible and the ability to meet them altered as necessary.

The only goals you have to worry about initially are the first ones you write down (or if you prefer, just summarize them in your head). Even if you just think of one goal and keep it in mind, that's a great start. Then at specific time intervals, perhaps every month, think of new goals. If you write your goals down, it's a good idea to post them somewhere that you'll see them (perhaps on the home page of your computer or on the refrigerator) or to make an index card that you carry with you.

If you don't meet one or more of your goals, this isn't a failure, rather it's a normal part of the process. Take the time to analyze why you didn't meet a particular goal and make appropriate adjustments to revise it. Florence Chadwick learned this when she decided to become the first woman ever to swim twenty-one miles across the Catalina Channel off the coast of California. For years she trained and then in 1952, she was finally ready to try. She began full of hope surrounded by people in small boats encouraging her to keep going. As she neared her goal, there was a heavy fog and the waters became increasingly cold and choppy. Finally, just a half mile from the coastline, she gave up and asked to be pulled into a boat. Florence was heartbroken and later said to reporters, "Look, I'm not excusing myself, but if I could have seen land I know I could have made it." Florence Chadwick, though defeated once, decided to try again. The second time around she concentrated on developing a mental image of the coast— her finish line. She had a goal and a clear vision of where she wanted to be at the end of her journey. This time she made it.

I'm often asked a very basic but extremely important question, which goes something like, "How do you get people to begin to heal when they are so sick and everything is a huge effort?" My answer is always that I don't "get" people to do anything. I may help to inform them and encourage them, but ultimately each person has to take responsibility for his or her own healing journey. However, what I have found is that once someone begins, the process becomes much easier and flows nicely.

You may be thinking that you simply can't add one more thing to your list of responsibilities. The idea of establishing goals may feel very overwhelming. So, before adding any new goals to your daily routine and letting these new responsibilities discourage you, consider two things. First, setting goals allows you to accomplish things that are important to you. Goals help you decide what are the most important things you should be concentrating on. What is most deserving of your time and attention as you go through this healing experience? The second thing is that you may find setting goals actually gives you more rather than less time. By choosing what to focus on, you are also making decisions about what is *not* a priority in your life right now. I often tell my patients that they have "permission" to avoid doing all the boring and physically tiring things they did before they were sick and can concentrate on what means the most to them—physically and emotionally.

The next chapter focuses on how to take the time to heal. Even if you feel a bit discouraged right now, by continuing to read you are going in the right direction on your healing journey. And, as the great physician and poet, Dr. Oliver Wendell Holmes once said, "The greatest thing in the world is not so much where we are, but in what direction we are moving."

chapter 3

Take the Time to Heal

One day, a woman in her seventies came to my office, and though she was very active, she rarely ventured more than a few miles from home. My office was a little over thirty miles from her house, and it had taken her more than an hour by car to get to her appointment. When I went in to see her, she told me that it was frustrating to drive so far to see a doctor, but she was happy to be seeing a specialist. On an impulse, I mentioned that some of my patients come from other countries to get their medical care in the United States. They have to deal with not only car rides, but long plane flights, delays in customs, checking into a hotel, and getting to a medical appointment in a foreign city. It's not easy, and yes, it takes them a lot of time.

Having some perspective about time is important. Healing takes time—usually more time than we want it to take. Taking time to heal can be a tremendous challenge as you struggle to balance "real life" with health priorities. Many people who are in the process of recovering feel as though they are in limbo—not able to live as they did before while simultaneously not able to devote all their time and energy to healing.

It would be nice to tell others, "I'm having my own crisis right now; let's schedule yours for another day." (Or better yet, let's not have any crises at all!) However, life doesn't work that way. Things happen to us and to our loved ones that need immediate attention. Sometimes, we find ourselves in the midst of more than one drama at a time. So, taking the time to heal doesn't mean that the real world disappears. Most of the time you will have to operate in two time zones.

It's not only a crisis that makes us pay attention to real world issues. As I was healing from toxic cancer treatments, the day-to-day challenges were always present. I was constantly frustrated thinking about whether I should focus on what I needed to do or what my children needed me to do. When I returned to work, I had even more challenges as I tried to finish healing while, at the same time, do my job. There isn't an easy solution for living in these two time zones, and I did what I had to do: I compromised. I tried to stay focused on my efforts to heal, but sometimes this went by the wayside as I lived my real life with real people who had immediate and pressing needs.

Of the thousands of seriously ill people I have treated, the one thing that nearly all of them want is more time. Sometimes, the stated goal of having more time needs a little translation. Often when people say they want more time, what they really want is more energy to accomplish the things they desire. Time and energy are interrelated and increasing one often enhances the other. In fact, time and energy are two of the most important commodities for everyone.

More than a century ago, Arnold Bennett wrote, *How to Live on 24 Hours a Day,* which became a bestseller in the United States and England. In the book, Bennett described time as "the ideal democracy" and wrote:

> In the realm of time there is no aristocracy of wealth, and no aristocracy of intellect. Genius is never rewarded by even an extra hour a day . . . the chief beauty about the constant supply of time is that you cannot waste it in advance . . . The next year, the next day, the next hour are lying ready for you, as perfect, as unspoilt, as if you had never wasted a single moment in all your career.

This is such an empowering way to look at the time that you have. Rather than worry about what you may have "wasted," focus on the fact that you have a new day with which to begin to achieve your goals.

I think of taking the time to heal as a literal "investment" in one's health. After all, for many people time is money and spending one's hours on physical and emotional recovery means that there is less money in the bank. However, it's a great investment. Think about how much it would be worth to you if you could upgrade your health. Chances are that you'd be willing to pay quite a lot. Many people would say that this commodity is priceless. Of course, you can't simply write a check and improve your health. But you can invest your time, and whatever other costs you may incur, in enhancing your health. Just as you would with any major life decision, it's important to think this through and then make a commitment to investing the time it will take to mend.

It's not easy to give yourself permission to take the time to heal. You probably have a lot of responsibilities and people counting on you. Taking the time to heal is a way of nurturing yourself. In turn, the more you nurture yourself, the better you can nurture others.

Make Healing a Priority

There is a story about a man who seeks enlightenment. He travels a great distance to consult a Zen master. The master invites the man to tea and fills his cup to the brim. Every time the man takes a drink, the master refills the cup to the point where it overflows onto the saucer. The master is silent all the while, and finally the man who is becoming increasingly exasperated, asks the master why he doesn't say anything but just keeps pouring tea. The master responds, "Your cup is too full. You keep adding to it and now it is overflowing. There is no room for enlightenment until you empty your cup." This is true of healing optimally as well. If your life is bursting at the seams, you won't have the time or the energy to recover as well as possible. You'll need to empty your cup a bit to make room to heal.

Making time to focus on healing can certainly be challenging, but one thing that really helps is to prioritize your daily activities. As you consider and plan your goals, keep in mind that you want to be devoting the maximum amount of time in your day to doing those things that will help you to heal. If you don't do this, and instead spend your time running your body into the ground by working too much or too hard or doing too many errands or chores, you will be both physically and emotionally exhausted, and you likely won't be able to heal optimally. You want to focus on what will give you energy and strength.

In order to reach your goals, you will need to use your emotional and physical reserves wisely. Healing is not about pushing yourself to the limit without consideration for what tasks are important or how they will affect your body. Rather, recovering well involves a thoughtful approach where you set goals and modify your activities to achieve those goals. While healing well does include physically challenging your body to improve your strength and endurance, it also involves periods of relaxation and rest—emotionally recharging. In short, in order to heal well, you need to make it a priority and begin to pace yourself.

Everyone has to prioritize their activities and pace themselves, but when you are focused on healing, this becomes particularly important. When I talk to my patients about these concepts, they often jump to the conclusion that I am telling them not to do the things they enjoy. In fact, that's not what I'm recommending. Instead, think of this as your chance to unload all of the boring and monotonous tasks that you never enjoyed doing anyway. This has been a societal trend for a number of years. We now have ways to order tickets to events without standing in line, to obtain groceries without ever going to the store, to get our clothes dry-cleaned by setting a bag filled with dirty garments outside our door, and so on. There are many ways to trim your to-do list while at the same time maintaining the time and energy to do what brings you pleasure.

Regardless of whether you decide to hire people or use various services to decrease your to-do list, this is a good time to let friends know how they can help. You certainly can do this in a very considerate way that will not overly burden those close to you. For example, inquire when your friend is next going shopping and ask whether he could pick up a short list of items for you at the same time. Or, request that a coworker pick up lunch for you when she goes out for a break. Also, if you consider what you did every day prior to your illness or injury, you'll likely find that there are plenty of things you did in the past which simply don't need to be done at all or at least not in the same way. For instance, while I would not suggest that anyone skip bathing altogether, changing from a daily shower to an every-other-day routine, is a great way to conserve energy.

At the end of the chapters in this book, I provide some Healing Strategies. Later in this chapter, Table 3.1 lists pacing principles that may be helpful to you. In Table 3.2, I include a healing strategy that encourages you to consider filling out a three-day log of your activities. This is something that I do with my patients, and it is a great way to see how you are spending your time and energy. It's important to match your goals to what you actually do every day. You can perform your own analysis. A three-day log is simple to do and it will help you figure out how to prioritize your activities and pace yourself as you recover.

Make Time for a New Beginning

Virginia Woolf once wrote an essay on being ill. She elegantly stated what many others have experienced—that illness, with all its inherent problems and changes, also provides opportunities. Woolf penned it this way: "Considering how common illness is, how tremendous the spiritual changes that it brings, how astonishing, when the lights of health go down, the undiscovered countries that are then disclosed . . ."

While there is no doubt that there are "undiscovered countries" to explore, this doesn't mean that illness bestows "gifts" (though some people think so, that was not my experience). I don't like to think of illness as something that bears gifts—I worry that this concept is overly simplified and may marginalize people and their profound experiences. However, it's a fact that all of our experiences provide opportunities. When you experience illness, it changes your life. It takes you down an alternate path and shows you places that are different from what you've seen before. Almost always, this path is dark and frightening. Always it is lonely, for the ill person ultimately travels alone.

As the darkness lifts and you begin to heal, there is opportunity and hope. A new beginning, not a chance to go back to the person you were before—that's not possible. Instead, this new beginning allows you to become the person you will be in the future—one who must incorporate this experience into the fabric of your life. It's helpful sometimes to recognize this new beginning for what it is: a turning point, a chance, a lifting of the "darkness."

Taking the time to heal is an investment in you, your family, and your future. It is the most valuable gift you can give yourself and your loved ones.

Healing Strategies

Table 3.1 Pacing Basics

There are a few basic principles when it comes to pacing. These may seem obvious, but as you read them ask yourself whether you are doing them. If not, they are good tools to use in the recovery process. The basics of pacing are as follows:

1. Organize and plan your day ahead of time.
Doing this costs you energy up front but is a very important thing to do. This goes back to priorities. Skip the things that aren't that meaningful or cause you to be overly fatigued. Include the activities that will help you with your recovery and those things which you enjoy. If you need to do something that you know will be tiring (such as painting your home, doing your taxes, and so on), spread it out over several days or even weeks. Better yet, ask someone else to do it for you. Try to exercise early in the day when your energy is highest. This won't work for everyone's schedule, and exercise is important to include even if you do it later in the day. Keep in mind that exercising right before bed can contribute to poor sleep.

2. Plan and take breaks (rest periods).
This doesn't mean that you should take a nap. I only recommend napping if you are sleeping well at night and still

exhausted during the day. If you aren't sleeping well at night and you nap during the day, this sets up a vicious cycle of poor sleep. Most people don't need to nap during the day and would do better with an earlier bedtime or a later wake-up time, or both. However, planning breaks during the day is important to give your body and your mind a rest. You should find time to sit down in a comfortable chair and read, listen to music, meditate—to do whatever you find relaxing. Depending on your energy level, stage of recovery, current treatment regimen, and work and family commitments, you may have to be creative in when and how you are able to take breaks. But, do it. Put your feet up and be good to yourself.

3. Use good body mechanics.
Poor body mechanics are a huge energy drain. Sitting at your computer in a chair that is not supportive and without arm rests (sometimes called data arms if they attach to the desk and are not part of the chair) is very taxing. Standing (and bending over) while doing household chores such as cooking, folding laundry, washing the car, and gardening is also very tiring. Don't mistake activities such as these for exercise. These tasks will do little to build your strength and endurance, so you should conserve your energy while performing them during healing.

4. Perform activities in comfortable temperatures.
I know some of my friends take great pride in waiting until a certain predetermined date to turn on their air-conditioning or

(cont'd)

heat, despite the outdoor temperature. It's great to be frugal and to be conscious of the environment. However, it takes a lot of extra energy for you to keep your body warm. Living or working in an environment that is too hot or too cold will unnecessarily sap your energy. It is also wise to avoid exercising in the extreme heat or cold.

5. Avoid straining or pushing yourself to the point of exhaustion.

I tell my patients to listen to the "voice" of their bodies. What is your body telling you? Are your legs or arms getting tired? Are you feeling more pain? Are you having trouble concentrating? These are all warning signs that you are pushing too hard. Try to heed these warning signs right away so that you don't reach the point of severe exhaustion, pain, or other discomfort.

Table 3.2 How to Fill Out a Three-Day Activity Log

To figure out what you are currently doing and how you might want to modify your activities, try spending three days keeping track of what you are doing and how you feel during the day. Write down all of your activities and also document when you are experiencing pain or feeling particularly fatigued. Use highlighters and rate each task as low, moderate, or high energy. For example, a yellow marker can highlight the low-energy activities, a pink marker can highlight activities that take a moderate amount of energy, and high-level activities can be in green. To rate pain and fatigue, use a scale from 0 to 10 (0 is when you have no pain or fatigue and 10 is severe pain or fatigue). It is really interesting and helpful to see how your log "lights up" and also what you are doing or just did that may relate to an increase in pain and/or fatigue. You'll get a lot of good information from this exercise if you have the patience to do it.

Step 1
Organize a notebook with space to write in for each hour of the day for three days.

Step 2
Record your activities each waking hour for the next three days.

(cont'd)

Step 3

As you record your activities, also write down when you have pain or feel fatigued. Rate pain and/or fatigue from 0 to 10.

Step 4

After your log is completed, take three different colored highlighters and mark each hour of activity as low, moderate, or high energy. It is really interesting and helpful to see how your log "lights up."

Step 5

Now, analyze your log. Are your activities well balanced, or is there too much of one color? When are you feeling particularly fatigued or in pain? Which activities are really important to you and which ones can you eliminate? What are you doing that is helping you to physically recover and what is hindering your ability to mend? Finally, as you look at your log and consider your goals, how do your daily activities match up with achieving what you consider your top priorities?

Heal Yourself from the Inside Out

chapter 4

You Can Use Your Mind to Heal

One day, I was doing a radio interview about what helps people heal, and the discussion was focused on how powerful the mind-body connection is. The man who was interviewing me startled me when he said, "I agree that the mind is really powerful. In fact, I think that people who are ill really want to be sick or they wouldn't be." His point was that since our thoughts influence our physical and emotional state, we could simply wish illness away. And, if we didn't wish it way, it's because we really want to remain sick. Needless to say, I disagreed with him on this point.

Healing yourself from the inside out begins by tapping into the powerful mind-body connection. This has been researched extensively, and your mind is perhaps your most powerful healing tool. However, it doesn't mean that just because you channel your thoughts a certain way, your body will instantly be healed. On the other hand, some people think that our thoughts and emotions really don't change our physical state. That's not true, either. They are very much interconnected and influence each other continuously.

I will admit that telling someone to simply think about being healed and it will happen sounds like magic, sorcery, or nothing short of a miracle. However, there's more to the mind-body relationship than wizardry or just a fantastic illusion. Your thoughts and emotions produce verifiable changes in your body, which influence its physical state, and vice versa. A classic example of this occurs when you run or exercise vigorously. While you are doing a physical activity, there are many chemical and biological reactions that are occurring in your body. Many people have described the "runner's high" or euphoric feeling they get after a long run. This is really the result of physical changes such as the release of endorphins that influence how good you feel. This might seem like a one-way reaction whereby if you do something good for your body, then it positively impacts your mind. However, the opposite is also true—studies show that your mind has the ability to improve your physical state through chemical and biological reactions that happen in your body.

For example, Dr. Herbert Benson, a Harvard cardiologist and notable pioneer in mind-body medicine, conducted many studies verifying how our brains can influence our bodies. He is internationally renowned and highly respected, and his work has led to considerable change within the scientific community about the importance of mind-body medicine in preventing and recovering from serious illness.

Dr. Benson is probably best known for his work on what he calls "the relaxation response." Few people who have studied the results of the relaxation response would doubt its effectiveness. This response, which I describe how to perform later in this chapter, is the opposite of the stress response commonly known as "fight or flight." In a stressful situation, the sympathetic nervous system goes into overdrive and increases heart rate, blood pressure, breathing rate, and blood supply to the muscles in order for the body to respond to stress. The relaxation response is the opposite of this and works by encouraging the parasympathetic nervous system to take over. Dr. Benson has shown that the relaxation response results in measurable and consistent physical changes including a decrease in blood pressure, heart and breathing rates, metabolism, and muscle tension. At the same time, some brain waves increase. There is an indisputable mind-body chain of reactions that takes place when people are able to perform the relaxation response.

Dr. Benson is not alone in researching the relationship between how we function physically and emotionally. In fact, many well-respected scientists began to study this in earnest during the latter part of the twentieth century, and in doing so pioneered a new field of medicine called psychoneuroimmunology. This area of research focuses on how our brains and bodies are interconnected and how this relationship affects health and disease. Dr. Benson and others who have dedicated their career to mind-body medicine have done so at great risk to their reputations. However, their courage and conviction have paid off and few people today would argue that this is all "hooey." Science writer Henry Dreher summed it up this way, "These explorers, leaders of such fields as psychoneuroimmunology, neuroimmunomodulation, and psychoneuroendocrinology, sneaked past the closed doors of biomedical compartmentalization with the fearlessness of cat burglars . . ."

Dreher explains in his book, *Mind-Body Unity,* that one reason why these "visionary mind-body scientists" have had so many public opinion obstacles to overcome is because mind-body medicine has often been reduced to the simplistic and quite detrimental slogan of "mind over matter." This is basically what the gentleman who interviewed me on the radio was suggesting. Mind-body medicine is not quite that simple, and reducing it to "if you think good thoughts, you'll be healed" is just not accurate. Dreher writes:

> Popular culture has enshrined the concept of a "mind-body connection," . . . [The] term reflects outdated ideas from the predecessor field of psychosomatic medicine, as well as rather simplified concepts that stem from today's broader culture of alternative medicine . . . (It is generally agreed among mind-body scientists that mind does not lord its putative powers over matter; rather, mind and matter are intertwined in a kind of dialectic dance.)

Many of the current areas of research in this field focus on mind-body therapies, such as meditation, imagery, prayer, relaxation, biofeedback, and hypnosis, and how they impact us physically. Though it is absolutely clear that there are numerous ways in which our brains affect our bodies and vice versa, this is not a simple concept where there is a linear relationship and a straightforward cause and effect result.

The best way to think about this is that the mind-body connection has to do with bidirectional chemical and biological reactions that influence your mental and physical health; however, neither your mind nor your body totally controls the other.

An outdated concept is the belief that all stress is harmful to us physically and results in a depressed immune system. This has been replaced with a better understanding of how stress can be helpful in some instances and harmful in others—depending on many factors, including how long the stress lasts, how severe it is, how well prepared in advance we are to handle it, and so on. The bottom line is that in this field of medicine, while we are certain that there is significant mind-body flow that is bidirectional, easily understood platitudes such as "all stress is bad" don't seem to hold up.

During the 1970s when the field of psychoneuroimmunology had not yet become well established, Dr. Norman Cousins wrote a famous book titled *Anatomy of an Illness as Perceived by the Patient*. In this book, he discussed many of the aspects of mind-body medicine and how they may affect health. However, there was very little research to support his claims and, not surprisingly, some experts regarded this book with a fair amount of skepticism. In summarizing the mind-body unity, Dr. Cousins wrote, "What we are talking about essentially . . . is the chemistry of the will to live." Decades later, scientists have studied mind-body medicine, and there is now significant research to support how your body and mind influence each other in a bidirectional manner and how this can positively affect your health.

Undoubtedly, there exists a powerful mind-body relationship. Though scientists are still investigating how it works, it's clear that we can take advantage of interventions that utilize our mind's healing forces. This is a sophisticated view of medicine that is based on much research and is really a "best of both worlds" scenario. Engaging your mind in the recovery process can help you to psychologically and physically heal as well as you possibly can.

Healing Strategies

To encourage your mind to heal your body, try one or more of these strategies:

Meditation

Set aside time each day to meditate, even if it's just for five to ten minutes. You can meditate longer (twenty to thirty minutes) as you develop your skill and it becomes more enjoyable. Find a comfortable but supportive place to sit. Your posture should be erect, but you want to feel at ease. You can have soft music playing or you can be in a public place with noise—it doesn't matter how loud it is, though it's easier to start meditating in a peaceful place. Plan to be present in the moment without any other agenda. Use your breathing to help keep your mind from wandering. At first, you will likely have a lot of intrusive thoughts; just gently push them away. Meditation gets easier the more you practice. Also, there are many good resources for learning to meditate, including books, audio CDs, apps, and the like.

Visualization and Imagery

In this technique, you concentrate on a specific vision or event. The theory behind this is that the mind is able to cure the body when visualized images evoke sensory memory, strong emotions, or fantasy. One image I particularly like is from a painted card that an artist friend and cancer survivor sent me. This card shows the image of a tree. If you look closely, you can see that the tree is also a woman. The two images are meshed together. On the back of this painting she wrote, "Strong as a tree—and reaching up—up to faith and surrounded by those who love her."

Many people will visualize more than one scene, sort of like a short film clip that you control. For example, you may visualize medicine flowing into your body and cancer cells flowing out of your body. Or, you may visualize your body working perfectly in concert toward a goal such as winning a race. Maybe you'll imagine you are at an event, such as a wedding, or on vacation, or swimming in the ocean. There are many ways to use visualization, but to get started, think about what is meaningful to you and use that as your vision.

Progressive Muscle Relaxation

In this technique, you either lie down or sit in a comfortable place and begin by tensing and then relaxing muscles throughout your body. Start at the top and grimace and clench your teeth. After counting to ten, relax, inhale, and exhale, and let your face be as lax as if you were asleep. Next, tense your neck and shoulders and count to ten. Relax again and repeat with your chest, abdomen, buttocks, arms, hands, legs, and feet.

Relaxation Response

In his book *The Relaxation Response,* Dr. Herbert Benson describes two essential steps to eliciting this response. They are:

1. Repetition of a word, sound, phrase, prayer, or muscular activity.
2. Passively disregarding everyday thoughts that inevitably come to mind and returning to your repetition.

In order to perform this technique, Dr. Benson suggests the following strategies:

1. Pick a focus word, short phrase, or prayer that is firmly rooted in your belief system.
2. Sit quietly in a comfortable position.
3. Close your eyes.
4. Relax your muscles, progressing from your feet to your calves, thighs, abdomen, shoulders, neck, and head.

5. Breathe slowly and naturally, and as you do, say your focus word, sound phrase, or prayer silently to yourself as you exhale.

6. Assume a passive attitude. Don't worry about how well you're doing. When other thoughts come to mind, simply say to yourself, "Oh well," and gently return to your repetition.

7. Continue for ten to twenty minutes.

8. Do not stand immediately. Continue sitting quietly for a minute or so, allowing other thoughts to return. Then, open your eyes and sit for another minute before rising.

9. Practice the technique once or twice daily. Good times to do so are before breakfast and before dinner.

The four mind-body strategies I describe here are safe and easy to do and can help you tap into your mind-body connection. If you are using one of them already, try adding another to your daily routine. Remember when you start a new strategy that it takes some time to get used to it. As you practice it, you will feel more comfortable and the mind-body strategy you are using will become more powerful in helping you to heal. I suggest getting started with at least one of the four I have described in this chapter; however, these are just suggestions. You can use whatever strategies feel comfortable to you.

chapter 5

You Can Use Self-Love to Heal

The impressive power of love is a potent "medicine" that can prevent illness before it strikes and help those who are stricken heal more quickly and completely. In fact, love can positively affect not only one's quality of life but also the quantity of one's days. This is why the well-regarded heart specialist, Dr. Dean Ornish, wrote an entire book on the healing power of love and intimacy. In this fascinating bestseller, which was published in 1998, aptly titled *Love and Survival,* Dr. Ornish writes, "If a new drug had the same impact, virtually every doctor in the country would be recommending it for their patients. It would be malpractice not to prescribe it . . ."

Indeed, the idea of using love as a healing strategy is appealing. But, does it really work? Can receiving love from yourself and from others help you to heal physically and emotionally? Absolutely. There is a chemical basis for love and many physiological consequences when love is given and received. In addition to this, loving yourself means that you listen to your healing voice, take the time to heal, and are motivated to work toward your goals.

Take Time to Nurture Yourself

Most of us are better at nurturing others than nurturing ourselves. For example, one day I was giving a speech at a cancer fund-raiser. This fund-raiser was at a hotel and included a "spa day" for attendees. When I talked to the women who came, all of them felt good about spending the money on pampering because it was, after all, going to a good cause. These same women, though, told me that they wouldn't normally take the time or spend the money to nurture themselves with facials, manicures, and massages. This spa day was on the "approved" list because its true purpose was to nurture others—people with cancer—not themselves.

Men and women, but particularly women according to the research, often do not learn the skill of self-nurture. Sigmund Freud considered self-nurture a form of narcissism that was infantile and pathologic. But times have changed, and we now understand that people who love themselves are much better at loving others than those who don't. Another way of saying this is that you will be better at nurturing those who need you if you nurture yourself first. A more modern look at narcissism and nurture involves having high self-esteem, which means that you value yourself and your health.

However, despite the shift that has taken place in the field of psychology over the concept of self-nurture, this hasn't necessarily translated into individuals becoming better at taking care of themselves. Harvard psychologist Alice

Domar wrote in her groundbreaking book, *Self-Nurture: Learning to Care for Yourself As Effectively As You Care for Everyone Else,* "The capacity to self-nurture starts with our relationship with our parents . . . As children, did we learn the value of self-love and self-care? Did our mothers and fathers present themselves as strong role models of self-nurturance, or were they ceaseless models of self-sacrifice, self-doubt, self-neglect, or even self-abuse?" While both men and women often lack the skills to nurture themselves, according to the research, women find it particularly difficult.

One of my patients, a woman I'll call Joan, is a classic example of someone who is terrific at nurturing others and not very good at taking care of herself. Joan recently had surgery for a low back problem. She took a short period of time off from work and then returned to a full-time position. At her follow-up appointment with me, she was in tears and said, "I thought I could handle this but I can't. I'm too weak." I was curious about what prompted Joan to go back to work so soon after her surgery. Her surgeon had advised her to take more time off, so I assumed that Joan was worried she'd lose her job or that her family needed her salary. Neither of these was the case. In fact, Joan told me that she was receiving her full salary and no one at work had put any pressure on her to return. Instead, as someone who constantly nurtured others, she had a hard time not being able to do this and decided to go back to her previous role at work. Joan told me that "people count on me," and she believed she should go back to work even though she didn't physically feel ready.

When I talked to Joan, she realized the people at work were getting along just fine without her. They missed her, of course, and when she was there they had less work to do. However, her colleagues were willing to support her during this time, and after our appointment Joan recognized that she needed to take the time to finish recovering so that she could go back to work and be productive and helpful. What Joan needed to do was to nurture herself, or what some psychologists have termed engage in a "healthy selfishness." Psychology professors Richard and Rachael Heller define healthy selfishness as "a way of thinking and acting in which there is a deep appreciation, compassion, and concern for yourself—by yourself. It includes (but is not limited to) your willingness to: respect your feelings, sensitivities, preferences, desires, and needs; trust your knowledge, ability, and experience; accept your weaknesses and imperfections without blame or guilt; encourage your effort and struggles, without demand for success; and offer unconditional love and nurturing of the child within." When you are healing, you need to focus on yourself in a loving and nurturing manner. At times, you'll want to put yourself first—what you need must take precedence over the needs of others. This isn't easy to do if you've been taught, as many of us have, that we should be more concerned with others than with ourselves.

Sometimes, it's easier to embrace self-nurturing if you consider the opposite option, self-denial. Drs. Heller and Heller define self-denial as "the surrendering of your needs, preferences, and desires in order to fulfill the needs, preferences, or desires of another person." Though chronic self-denial is unhealthy, it is particularly problematic if you are recovering from a serious illness or injury. This is truly a time when your focus should first and foremost be on helping yourself to heal.

If you find it difficult to take the time to nurture yourself, you are in good company. Many wonderful people are not good self-nurturers. Nevertheless, it's important to try and change this a bit as you mend. Begin with small steps. There is no doubt that illness provides opportunities, and one of those is a chance to reflect on how to take better care of yourself.

Of course, great excuses are plentiful: I don't have time. I keep forgetting. I'll do it later. I *am* going to do it—but not yet. The best excuse of all is, "Taking care of myself is not as important as all the other things I have to do—for other people. . . ."

I can't tell you how to balance your responsibilities in the time zones of real life and recovery, but I can encourage you to simply do the best that you can. Try to stay focused on healing, but at the same time recognize that it's okay to take some breaks and do what you need to do in the real world. Keep in mind that the better you heal and the more strength and energy you have, the easier it will be for you to resume your former responsibilities and care for those who depend on you. As Shakespeare noted in *Henry V*, "Self-love, my liege, is not so vile a sin, as self-neglecting."

Healing Strategies

Table 5.1 Ways to Nurture Yourself

Listen to music, a nature sounds CD, audiobooks, or a relaxation
   tape

Meditate or pray

Watch television

Read a book or magazine

Sit down and talk to someone in person or on the phone

Perform deep breathing and relaxation exercises

Play a game on the computer or a card game by yourself or
   with a friend

Play a musical instrument

Crochet, macramé, knit, needlepoint, or sew

Make a craft or jewelry

Carve wood

Scrapbook

Do a jigsaw or crossword puzzle

Draw or paint a picture

Write a letter, e-mail, journal entry, poem, or short story

Sit in a comfortable place with a warm drink (decaffeinated
   and nonalcoholic is best)

Lie down and take time to reflect

Go for a scenic drive

Sit outside or take a walk someplace where you can enjoy nature

Go for a manicure, pedicure, massage, or other spa treatment

Exercise

chapter 6

You Can Lessen Your Emotional
Pain to Heal

There is no doubt that in healing, mood matters. Research studies have demonstrated a great deal about how our mood may affect healing. There are three key points that deserve some explanation. The first point is that *your mood specifically influences chemicals in your body that have a direct effect on physical healing.*

Though the relationship between our emotions and their effect on our bodies is as old as mankind, only recently have scientists begun to study this field in earnest. As I mentioned earlier, this research is compelling and contributes to the field of psychoneuroimmunology, the study of how what we experience psychologically affects us physically, especially the brain and nervous and immune systems. This area of medical research has shown how stress and other emotions affect healing.

For example, stress is a reliable predictor of delayed wound healing and seems to "age" our bodies prematurely.

A now classic study done in 1998 on stress and wound healing involved a group of healthy dental student volunteers who underwent placement of wounds in their mouths on two occasions. During the first round, the wounds were timed during summer vacation. The second-round wounds was timed three days before the first major examination of the term. Not surprisingly, the wounds planted before the exam took 40 percent longer to heal. The researchers concluded, "These data suggest that even something as transient, predictable, and relatively benign as examination stress can have significant consequences for wound healing."

A different study that looked at whether relieving stress would help facilitate wound healing involved another group of healthy volunteers who received an identical wound in the upper arm. Thirty-six people participated and they were divided into two groups. One group, half of the volunteers, were asked to write about an emotional event in their lives, preferably one they had not talked about much before. The other group wrote about trivial matters. In this study, those participants who wrote about the traumatic events healed faster, which lead researchers to conclude that relieving stress by writing about it is helpful in physical recovery.

In both of these studies, investigators were looking at healthy volunteers and superficial wounds. However, researchers have recently been studying the relationship between stress and wound healing in people who are recovering from surgical incisions. In one study evaluating psychological stress and wound healing in people recovering from a hernia repair operation, researchers found that "greater worry" predicted lower levels of matrix metalloproteinase-9 in the wound fluid (these proteins can be measured and are known to help facilitate tissue regeneration and healing), more painful wounds, and delayed healing.

Perfect Control Is Not Possible

There is clearly a strong link between physical healing and our emotions. Though the scientific research is convincing that mood matters when it comes to physical healing, it's unrealistic to think that we can tightly control our feelings at an incredibly emotional time in our lives.

This brings me to my second point: *It is impossible to perfectly control your mood—especially while you are focusing on healing and so much is happening to you both physically and emotionally.* Bad moods, grief, and worry are all part of everyday life. Certainly, mood fluctuations may be more pronounced when someone is in need of healing. However, even during difficult times, it's important to temper one's emotions with periods of hope and optimism. I realize that it's much easier to write these words than to live them. It can be extremely difficult to give up the life you had planned in order to live the life you are faced with right now. But, there is no alternative, and healing as well as you possibly can allows you the possibility of having the future you want—even if it's altered from what you thought it would be.

Because this book focuses on how you can help yourself, I have limited this chapter to the kinds of emotional fluctuations that don't necessarily need medical intervention. However, it is not uncommon for people who are recovering to experience more profound emotional problems such as major depression, generalized anxiety disorder, or Post-Traumatic Stress Disorder (PTSD), which will require professional help and may include counseling and treatment with antidepressants or other medications. I have highlighted each of these conditions in Table 6.1. Talk to your doctor if you are experiencing symptoms of any of them.

With trauma or a new diagnosis such as cancer, people often experience a period of shock followed by grief. In *Good Grief,* former University of Chicago medicine and religion professor Granger Westberg wrote, "God has so made us that we can somehow bear pain and sorrow and even tragedy. However, when the sorrow is overwhelming, we are sometimes temporarily anesthetized in response to a tragic experience. We are grateful for this temporary anesthesia, for it keeps us from having to face grim reality all at once."

I'll never forget a young woman I treated while I was working at a military hospital during my residency. In a fit of anger, fueled by alcohol, this soldier got behind the wheel of a car and ended up colliding with a tree while driving at high speed. Thankfully, she survived this horrific accident, but her arm was so severely injured that it required an amputation. The young doctors I was working with at the time were all amazed at how accepting she seemed of this disfiguring and disabling injury. The older physicians, our mentors and teachers, wisely advised us that there would undoubtedly come a time when she would fiercely grieve.

They were right. What we saw initially, and this lasted for weeks, was a period of shock in which she was emotionally "anesthetized." She never cried and never appeared sad. Later, she did grieve and cried hard, racking sobs that resonated throughout the hospital corridors. Although it was painful to hear her grieve, she needed to mourn her arm and her altered life. (Refer to Table 6.2 for a list of the symptoms of grief versus depression.)

It is not uncommon for people to try to avoid mourning a loss—especially if it's a personal loss such as what can occur with illness or injury. Some people view grieving about themselves as an act of selfishness, though it certainly is not. Others who are deeply religious may deem grieving as akin to having a lack of faith. Westberg addresses this concern in his book and writes:

> Faith plays a major role in grief of any kind. But not in the way some people think. They often seem to have the idea that a person with strong faith does not grieve and is above this sort of thing. Moreover, these people imply that religious faith advocates stoicism. They might even quote the two words from Scripture, "Grieve not!" They forget to quote the rest of the phrase in which these two words are found: "Grieve not as those who have no hope" (1 Thessalonians 4:13).

Sociologist Arthur Frank has twice experienced life-threatening illness—once when he had a heart attack at thirty-nine-years of age, and the other just months after his heart attack, when he was diagnosed with testicular cancer. His reflections on illness include thoughts on mourning:

> These losses of future and past, of place and innocence, whether they are ours together or mine alone, must all be mourned. The ill person's losses vary according to one's life and illnesses. We should never question what a person chooses to mourn. One person's losses may seem eccentric to another, but the loss is real enough, and that reality deserves to be honored.

There's a storybook that I used to read to my children about a girl bear whose world is colorful and happy. The pages depict this lovely view of her surroundings. Seeing that she is not a cautious bear, however, her mother one day tells her that the world is filled with strangers and she mustn't talk to them. Suddenly, her worldview changes and the pages, depicting exactly what they showed before this discussion, are now darker and more menacing. I often thought of this book during my illness. I longed for the more colorful and lighthearted world I had inhabited, but I was stuck with a darker and more frightening world—at least for a time. At the end of the story, the young bear has more perspective and though her world is altered a bit, it's still a wonderful place.

Storybook endings are usually happily ever after, but the real world can be less kind. One of the reasons that this time in your life may be emotionally difficult is because of uncertainty about your recovery. While physical recovery

can be a bit unpredictable, you may find comfort in knowing that in terms of psychological healing, most people will
return to their usual emotional baseline after a period of
time. This is usually a gradual process and not one that you
can completely control. I remember the shock of my cancer
diagnosis and then a period of intense grieving while I ad-
justed to my new illness and wondered whether my prognosis would turn out to be very grave. Following this, my
emotions fluctuated, but overall they were more blunted
than usual. Not in the way that shock anesthetizes one initially, but in a more subtle way. I wasn't depressed, but I
certainly didn't feel as happy and optimistic as I usually do.
I was in a sort of emotional "no man's land." It reminded me
of the children's nursery rhyme:

> When you're up, you're up
> And when you're down, you're down
> But when you're only half way up,
> You're neither up nor down.

This blunting of emotions is normal and may last for
weeks or months as you work to physically and emotionally
recover. Healing is a process that sometimes moves forward,
sometimes loses ground, and still other times feels as though
you are stuck somewhere in the middle.

Your emotions may also be off-kilter because of chemical changes in your body from your illness or injury or due
to side effects from the treatments you are undergoing. Pain
medications and sleep drugs can sometimes paradoxically

worsen one's mood. "Cluster symptoms," such as fatigue, pain, poor sleep, depression, and anxiety, often are present to varying degrees in people who are physically healing. These symptoms not only can be found together but they can directly influence each other. For example, someone in pain may not sleep well and this will lead to fatigue. Then, constant fatigue and pain can contribute to feelings of sadness and even depression. This can be a vicious cycle, and recognizing it is the first step to breaking it.

Throughout your journey, the "real world" will also influence your emotions. Daily stress is inevitable and stems from many sources. I recall a conversation with a neighbor boy who was eleven years old at the time. He said, "I can't wait to be a grown-up because then I won't have so much stress!" I asked him about the things in his life that were currently stressful; he listed a host of daily trials and tribulations such as not having enough time to play and having too much homework. While his worries might seem trivial against the backdrop of serious illness, they are really a reflection of what everyone goes through, regardless of age. Small annoyances and aggravations are a constant presence in all of our lives.

Along with these daily irritations, we sometimes experience a more significant source of stress. Shortly after I finished chemotherapy and almost immediately after I returned to work part-time, a former colleague began to stalk me. As is true for many victims of stalkers, I didn't exactly know why I became a target. What I surmise is that this man, who I had worked with many years earlier (our previous relationship was superficially friendly, and we had been colleagues who briefly chatted on various occasions), had developed some type of serious psychiatric disorder. When he contacted me after several years of not communicating, we had a short conversation that seemed normal enough. He told me he was relocating and wanted to talk to me about seeking employment in the Boston health community. I agreed to meet with him.

When he came to my office, I sensed almost immediately that something was wrong, but I couldn't really discern what it was. Nevertheless, I truthfully told him that there weren't any positions open at my hospital for which he would be qualified. I ended the meeting quickly and wished him well. Unfortunately, his behavior only grew stranger after our meeting and he began coming to my workplace unannounced and would spend hours sitting across the street at the local Starbucks. He sent me strange e-mails, called my home and office, and generally acted like a stalker. The security people at my hospital had escorted him out on at least one occasion and had given him a formal written notice that if he returned, he would be trespassing.

Finally, I called the police. A detective came to see me and I explained the situation; I told him that my staff and I all felt uncomfortable, and that I didn't know this stalker's potential for violence. Not surprisingly, there wasn't a lot that the detective could do. However, he assured me that he would try to track down this man and strongly urge him to cease contacting me.

Obviously, this situation was incredibly stressful, and though I wanted to tell the police officer that stress wasn't good for me as I was trying to heal (I doubt he had any idea I had been ill, though I had the telltale sign of extremely short hair following complete hair loss during chemotherapy), I remained silent on that point and simply let him do his job. A few days later, the detective arrived unannounced at my office to tell me that he had tracked down my stalker and had strongly discouraged him from bothering me. While the stalking didn't immediately stop, I think this did dampen my former colleague's enthusiasm for contacting me and eventually he did stop.

Healing doesn't occur in a vacuum and real life stressors, whether they are minor or not, have an impact. So, an important question is, "If I feel stressed, worried, or sad, can I use this to my advantage? Yes, perhaps counterintuitively, you can use negative emotions to help you heal.

Negative Emotions Can Help You Heal

Though this may seem a bit counterintuitive, my third and final point is: *Negative emotions are an inevitable part of your journey and while an abundance of them can hamper physical recovery, you can use them to your advantage to help motivate you as you heal.*

Psychiatrist Jimmie Holland has described what she calls the "tyranny of positive thinking." Dr. Holland writes:

> The present-day tyranny of positive thinking sometimes victimizes people . . . Trying to get you to "put on a happy face," to pretend you are feeling confident when in fact

you are feeling tremendously fearful and upset, can have a downside. By feigning confidence and ease about your illness and its treatment, you may cut off help and support from others. You may also be hiding anxious and depressed feelings that could be alleviated if you told your doctor how you really feel.

There are strategies that you can use to "tune in" to your emotions and monitor and even improve how you feel as you mend. As you consider how you feel, keep in mind that while *stress breeds more stress,* this doesn't mean that endless worrying about your emotions is a good idea. Aiming to be appropriately concerned about your emotional state is the goal. So, in order to avoid being overly concerned about your mood and how it may be fluctuating, remember that worry and stress can be great motivators and can help you to focus on healing.

In *After Cancer Treatment: Heal Faster, Better, Stronger,* I wrote about how frightening a cancer diagnosis is and how while there is no way to eliminate one's fears, we can use them to help motivate us to heal. I wrote:

> There is no doubt that cancer is a worrisome diagnosis, regardless of what your prognosis is. We didn't choose cancer, cancer chose us. . . . This is one adventure that I would much rather have skipped, but I had no choice. Now all I can do is move forward with my life as a cancer survivor. I don't think that any of us in this ever-growing club, which initiates unwilling members, is completely

fearless. I wish that I could take away any fear that you have. I wish that I could eliminate my own fears. But I know I can't. Instead, what I suggest is to use whatever fear you have as a means of motivating yourself to do the best job that you can to heal. If you have to live with demons, make them work for you. Make them part of the healing process.

By far, my greatest inspiration comes from my patients and those individuals I have met through my work who have dealt with tremendous adversity—cancer as well as other serious illnesses and injuries. I have profound admiration for those who I have watched live through some truly devastating injuries and illnesses and who seemingly handle their health challenges with grace. I have been an earnest student learning from them for many years. One of these individuals is Trisha Meili, a beautiful young woman, who was raped and beaten. Today, her outward appearance, soft voice, and ready smile give very little indication of her enormous suffering. However, on April 19, 1989, when she arrived in the emergency room, she had been brutally beaten. She had multiple fractures and her body temperature was eighty-five degrees. She was comatose and had lost so much blood that the doctors gave her little hope of surviving. Yet, she did survive this horrific ordeal after a long recovery period. You probably know Trisha as the Central Park Jogger. In her memoir, Trisha wrote, "I built a life until I was twenty-eight, was struck down, and so had to build another. Two lives, and I'm proud of both."

We can't completely control our emotions, but it's easy to think we can. There are many factors that play into how we feel at any given time. As you work to mend, you'll heal better if you spend some time taking care of your mental health. Physical and psychological health are undeniably linked. The more you improve physically, the better you feel emotionally and vice versa. This is a key part of "holistic" recovery—healing the "whole" body.

Healing Strategies

Consider your sources of stress and worry. What can you do to lessen them?

1.   Don't worry about worrying. One of the most important things you can do for yourself is not to worry about having too much stress or about the normal fluctuations in your mood. Worrying about worrying is not helpful.

2.   Tackle genuine sources of stress by figuring out a plan. In the case of my stalker, I had to go through formal channels that involved police intervention. Though I couldn't just get rid of this source of stress, it gave me comfort to take the necessary and appropriate steps to change the situation.

3.   Actively try to reduce day-to-day small levels of stress by implementing some strategies such as meditation. Table 6.3

lists simple things you can do to feel more relaxed and at peace.

4.   Recognize a more serious mood disorder. Review Table 6.1 to see if you may have a mood problem that needs medical attention.

5.   Treat yourself as a cherished friend. One of the best things you can do is to be kind to yourself. This means not being overly judgmental about your mood. There are plenty of "bad days" for everyone. It may help you to know that research on resilience and happiness shows that we often "overcatastrophize" about how bad something will be and then underestimate our ability to handle it. One study that highlights this tendency was done in the 1970s and looked at the happiness levels of three groups of people: (1) *lottery winners* who had won as much as one million dollars within the past year (the equivalent of tens of millions of today's dollars); (2) *motor vehicle accident victims* who were paralyzed after their injury; and (3) *control subjects,* regular Joes and Josephines from the same neighborhoods as the other two groups. As you may have guessed, the happiest group was the lottery winners, next came the regular Joes and Josephines, and in the rear were the folks who were paralyzed. However, the surprising part of this study was that the happiness of the individuals in these groups wasn't a lot different. The wealthy lottery winners were just slightly happier than the regular Joes and Josephines. The accident victims were close behind both groups—despite tremendous adversity.

This study confirmed what other research has shown, that people tend to be very resilient—even when faced with serious illness or injury.

6. Feed your brain healthy, upbeat messages. Are the messages and images you hear and see ones of hope and optimism or are they ones of tragedy and despair? As I went through cancer treatment, I realized how difficult it was for me to read the newspaper or listen to the news. The saying "If it bleeds it leads" is true. News media outlets are notorious for getting our emotions stirred up in a very negative manner. I'm not telling you to be ill informed about current events, but rather to consider what you are watching and listening to. This also goes for the books you read, the movies you watch, and even the people you talk to. How much of the information you are feeding your brain is hopeful, fun, and positive? Too much drama, whether it's fact or fiction, is not good for any of us. Therefore, as you ponder your mood goals, keep in mind that you want to move toward constantly giving your brain messages that are fortifying, heartening, and encouraging.

Table 6.1 Mood Problems that May Need Medical Intervention

Problem
Depression
Anxiety
Post-Traumatic Stress Disorder (PTSD)

Depression
Losing interest in usual activities and pastimes
Feeling irritable
Crying frequently
Feeling sad
Feeling hopeless
Having a poor appetite or significant weight loss
Having an increased appetite or significant weight gain
Sleeping poorly
Sleeping too much
Feeling agitated or restless
Feeling unusually fatigued
Having difficulty concentrating
Having difficulty making decisions
Feeling self-critical
Feeling excessively guilty
Feeling worthless
Having recurrent thoughts of dying or suicidal thoughts

Anxiety
Feeling tense or nervous
Feeling jittery or jumpy
Having difficulty relaxing
Feeling fatigued
Having muscle aches
Feeling restless
Feeling apprehensive
Feeling fearful or anticipating misfortune
Feeling sweaty or having clammy hands
Feeling chest palpitations or heart racing
Having a stomachache
Feeling light-headed or dizzy
Having difficulty sleeping
Feeling "on edge"
Feeling terrified without apparent reason
Anticipating impending doom
Feeling short of breath
Experiencing a choking or smothering sensation
Feeling faint
Trembling or shaking

Post-Traumatic Stress Disorder (PTSD)

Mental flashbacks

Startled by loud noises

Anxiety or depression

Poor sleep

Difficulty with concentration

Nightmares

Irritability

Anger

Table 6.2 Symptoms of Grief versus Depression

Grief

Sleep disturbances, changes in appetite, decreased ability to concentrate, less interest in social activities, alterations in usual behavior patterns (for example, more irritable or angry)

Generally waxes and wanes and people vacillate between feeling hopeful and sad; still able to enjoy activities

Depression

Similar symptoms as with grief but also may feel hopeless, helpless, worthless, guilty, and in some instances may have thoughts of suicide

Constant feelings of intense sadness, which affects most or all aspects of life; unable to enjoy activities

Table 6.3 Practical Things You Can Do to Reduce Stress and Improve Your Mood

Limit or avoid alcohol

Eat a well-rounded diet that is low in fat and high in fruits and vegetables

Get proper rest

Share your feelings with trusted family members, friends, or clergy

Consider joining a support group or contact some of the resources in the appendix for support

Exercise regularly

Practice meditating or imagery to help with relaxation

Commune with nature

Pray or tap into the Universe, if you are comfortable with this

Consider trying acupuncture

Consider having a massage or a manicure

Educate yourself about your diagnosis and how you can best help yourself

Keep a journal

Preserve routines that are comforting

Surround yourself with "feel-good" media (for example, books, television, and movies)

Continue hobbies that give you pleasure

Set limits with family, friends, and coworkers about what you are able to do

Combat frustration and sad feelings with positive outlets that help you focus on healing such as exercise, getting together with friends, and performing favorite hobbies

Avoid self-blame

Table 6.4 Physical Risk Factors that Can Contribute to Emotional Problems

Hormone imbalances
Nerve transmitter imbalances
High calcium levels
Anemia
Nutritional deficiencies
Poor sleep
Adrenal gland problems
Thyroid problems
Sodium or potassium imbalances
Medication side effects
Uncontrolled pain

Table 6.5 What to Discuss with Your Doctor

Any of the anxiety or depressive symptoms listed in Table 6.1
    that you are having
Any problems relating to sleeping well
Persistent pain
Unusual or persistent fatigue
Difficulty with exercise
Medication review to see if any might be contributing to mood
    disturbances (include everything you are taking—even if it
    is a nonprescription drug or a supplement)
Whether you might have a hormonal, nutritional, or other chem-
    ical imbalance

chapter 7

You Can Relieve Your Physical Pain to Heal

One day, I was driving with my two daughters. They were in the backseat, having an interesting conversation about pain. It went like this:

> "I have three Band-Aids on my body. One I have on my knee from when I fell down. Another one is from the splinter that Mom had to take out. The third one is where the nurse gave me a shot."

> "Oh yeah, well, I have a Band-Aid from the shots, too. Plus, I had to have my braces tightened and that *really* hurts."

> "Well, remember last night I had a headache?"

> "I've had a headache before, too!"

And on it went . . .

* * *

Pain is a nearly constant companion throughout our lives. As children, we all had the kinds of painful conditions that my daughters described. These pains, though bothersome, are fleeting and not terribly severe. However, serious illness can involve a much more intense and long-lasting pain experience. It can also involve discomfort that occurs due to a variety of reasons including the illness or injury itself, uncomfortable medical procedures, and side effects from medications. Just because I know a lot about treating pain doesn't mean that I didn't experience quite a bit of it. Pain is something that is almost always a part of serious illness and trying to eliminate all of it is generally not possible— nor is it necessarily a good idea.

How Pain Affects Healing

Physical discomfort can affect every aspect of someone's life, including sleep, physical activity, and diet. Beginning in the 1930s, ongoing studies have shown that sleep deprivation makes healthy volunteers more sensitive to pain. In one study of more than five hundred people who had undergone heart surgery between one and three years earlier, nearly one out of four participants reported chronic pain that was not cardiac in origin (angina). Of those who reported postoperative pain, almost 40 percent said that it interfered with their general activity level and with sleep. The researchers involved in this study commented, "When patients with and without chronic postoperative pain were compared, the former group had significantly higher levels of anxiety and depression, and they perceived their health-related quality of life as more compromised."

Studies reveal that pain has a direct physical connection to healing, and it also can cause emotional upheaval. There is no doubt that physical discomfort can cause enormous anxiety in people who have had serious heart problems. Worrying about "the next heart attack" is a legitimate concern, though very often the prognosis is excellent following surgery. Moreover, while musculoskeletal pain is common after cardiac surgery due to surgical incisions, this can still wreak havoc with the emotions of someone who has experienced a serious heart condition in the past. This kind of worry is also present in many other people who have experienced serious illness, including cancer survivors.

In many people who have suffered from a serious illness or injury that is associated with pain, there is something I call a "new pain filter." What I mean by this is that they begin to recognize pain in a new way and filter it through their brains differently than they did before they were ill. In someone who has had cancer, he or she might immediately react to nearly every pain sensation with the thought, "Maybe my cancer is back." In someone who has had a heart attack, any sort of sensation in the middle of the body may cause extreme worry. Frequently people who have had back or neck surgery come to my office, more concerned about needing "another surgery" than with whatever discomfort they are experiencing.

To fine-tune your pain filter, consider the following:

1. If you have a known current or past medical issue and either new or unchecked symptoms, see your doctor about this. You may need a medical workup or, at the least, some reassurance about whatever it is that you are experiencing.

2. Pain that is new, unidentified, or severe, and occurs in the chest, abdomen, or head should be investigated as soon as possible. This type of physical discomfort may indicate a serious problem that needs immediate medical attention.

3. Pain that is accompanied by other symptoms such as numbness, weakness, and dizziness should be investigated as soon as possible.

4. Physical discomfort that is caused by trauma should be attended to immediately (for example, after a car accident or a fall from a ladder), regardless of whether there is actual bleeding or other visible injury.

5. Most pain that people experience is musculoskeletal in origin. Musculoskeletal discomfort, such as that affecting the extremities, neck, and low back (muscular strains, tendonitis, arthritis, and so on), is usually not terribly serious—which is why a general rule to follow is to wait two weeks to see if the pain disappears. Persistent discomfort should not necessarily alarm you, but rather prompt you to seek out an appropriate diagnosis and treatment.

6.   As you fine-tune your pain filter, remember that serious pain usually declares itself—in other words, it's hard to ignore. For example, cancer pain is not typically intermittent. It doesn't usually come and go and wax and wane to a great degree. Rather, tumors that grow to the point where they are painful are pressing on structures that elicit pain. They often cause night pain and awaken people from sleep. The discomfort doesn't tend to change or go away for periods of time. Instead, cancer pain is the kind of persistent aching that makes you take notice. Though not all pain feels the same, discomfort that heralds a serious medical condition is usually hard to ignore.

7.   A doctor who can assess the problem and order appropriate tests should evaluate any pain that you experience.

While it's certainly understandable that people who have had a heart attack or cancer might be quite concerned about any uncomfortable sensations they are experiencing, *un*treated or *under* treated pain can also slow or impair healing in many other circumstances. For example, I distinctly recall a conversation I had with a woman who had recently undergone a total knee replacement surgery. She said, "If I could just sleep through the night, I could handle the pain during the day." Her words turned out to be a medically sound assessment. In a study that later came out, researchers noted that knee replacement surgeries were fairly standardized yet the outcomes in terms of pain and disability were quite variable. They found that higher levels of pain interfered with sleep and predicted poorer functional out-comes three months after surgery. The authors concluded, "The present findings underscore the importance of ade-quate sleep during postsurgical recovery and suggest that interventions targeting sleep disruptions may improve the speed and quality of patients' recovery from [total knee re-placement] and other surgical procedures." Which means, pain that interferes with sleep can affect the speed and com-pleteness of recovery.

It probably makes sense to you that pain can affect achieving a good night's sleep. Even if you don't awaken from pain, it can make your sleep restless and of poorer quality. There are several theories about how pain specifically affects sleep, with the first being what I just stated—that it aug-ments arousals. Another theory is that pain and sleep share common biological pathways—including the serotonergic system, which regulates serotonin and other chemical reac-tions in the body that may affect mood, pain, appetite, and so on. A third theory is that poor sleep can interfere with the way that we process pain—meaning that if you don't sleep well, you become more sensitive to discomfort. Each of these theories may play a role or one may someday be found to have more significance than the others. What is clear is that sleep and pain have a strong relationship to each other.

This is a classic good-news-bad-news situation. The bad news is that pain makes sleep worse and poor sleep in-creases the level of discomfort we experience. The good news is that improving sleep helps with alleviating pain and vice versa—another healing strategy that you can use to your advantage.

Depression (or anxiety) can also affect both pain and sleep. Persistent discomfort and depressed mood are commonly present together. For example, in a study examining depressive symptoms after a whiplash injury, the investigators found that of the approximately five thousand injured individuals, just over 42 percent developed depressive symptoms by six weeks after their injury. Another nearly 20 percent developed a depressed mood within a year after the whiplash. Not surprisingly, persistent pain combined with poor sleep tends to make people feel depressed. This cluster of symptoms—pain, fatigue, and depression—can hamper a person's ability to recover. On the other hand, addressing any one of these symptoms can lead to improvements in the others. Ideally, it's a good idea to work on goals that affect all of them—this will help to achieve optimal healing.

Take Steps to Relieve Your Pain

Pain is a symptom that needs to be explored—the right diagnosis is essential.

Physical discomfort can result from many different sources as one heals. It is absolutely critical when treating any discomfort to try and identify the cause. A man whom I will call Ken is a polio survivor who has quite a bit of residual paralysis but is able to walk. Though he's only in his late forties, his hip and knee joints have prematurely aged due to the fact that he doesn't have strong muscles that support his body and protect his joints. One day, he called my office and requested an appointment because his hip was hurting. When I saw him, he told me that I had "miraculously" cured his pain in the past and he was hoping for a similar "miracle" this time.

Ken had already seen his orthopedist who took an X-ray of his aching hip and told him that he likely will need to have a hip replacement because the arthritis was severe. However, when I questioned Ken and then examined him, rather than having the typical arthritic hip pain that radiates to the groin, he had lateral aching directly over a bursa (a fluid-filled sac that helps protect the hip joint). I told Ken I thought his symptoms were due to bursitis rather than arthritis and that a corticosteroid injection would do far more to alleviate his pain than a hip replacement. He agreed to try the injection, which I did that day. A couple of days later he sent me an e-mail stating the aching had indeed "miraculously" disappeared. Though Ken was incredibly relieved not to have any more hip pain (and delighted that he didn't need to have surgery), this is not due to a miracle but rather a simple case of making the right diagnosis.

If you are experiencing significant discomfort it's important to talk to your doctor about your symptoms and to accurately explain where the pain is located, how severe it is (you can use a numeric scale where 10 is intolerable and 0 is no pain at all), when it occurs, what makes it better or worse, what it feels like (for example, sharp or stabbing), whether it awakens you at night, and any associated symptoms (numbness, tingling, and so on).

This goes back to the concept of listening to what your body is telling you and not simply ignoring uncomfortable symptoms. At the same time, it's important to avoid jumping to conclusions that may not be accurate.

Pain can be treated in many different ways, and it is often a combination of treatments that work best.

There are many, many ways to treat pain; however, in general the treatments can be broken down into several categories. "Conservative" management is usually the first-line treatment and it works well for many problems. Conservative treatment means that the prescribed therapies are not "invasive." Invasive therapies are things such as injections or surgery. Conservative treatments may include (but are not limited to) using medications, ice or heat modalities, or physical and occupational therapy. Injections and surgery are sometimes first-line treatments for pain conditions (for example, in acute appendicitis, surgery is the appropriate treatment from the start), but in most cases conservative therapies are tried first.

My mother is a very nurturing person who frequently asks me to help out with the various ailments of her friends and acquaintances. Mom has two daughters who are doctors—my sister, Laura, is a pediatrician. We good-naturedly divide up her queries into two groups—Laura gets the calls about kids, and I get the calls about adults. I am always happy to assist if the problem is within the area of my expertise.

On one occasion, my mom, a former teacher, asked me to call her friend who happens to be a very dear woman who was my sixth-grade teacher. This woman was complaining of an ache in her shoulder due to a problem with her rotator cuff, which was so severe that she was not leaving her home. She had an appointment scheduled with her doctor the following week but was suffering terribly in the interim. I called her and asked her some questions and quickly found out that she was taking a combination of over-the-counter medication with a relatively low dose of two medications—ibuprofen and acetaminophen.

While she was concerned that she might need to have surgery, I reassured her that there were many things to try prior to giving this option serious thought. To start, I suggested she try a larger dose of straight ibuprofen three times a day and to alternate this with acetaminophen in between doses of the anti-inflammatory drug. Combination medications often provide too low of a dose of any single drug to effectively treat pain (refer to Table 1 for a list of commonly prescribed pain medications). Next, I recommended that she ice her shoulder three times a day for twenty minutes. Finally, I told her that physical therapy may be necessary, but she should check with her doctor. Basically, my advice boiled down to using a combination of conservative therapies simultaneously to achieve the best results (refer to Table 2 for a list of nonpharmacologic pain therapies). A week later my mom sent me an e-mail that said she and her friend, who was feeling much better, went out to dinner and had a wonderful time. Though this woman's pain was reduced, it is still possible that in the future she may benefit from other interventions such as an injection. However, the first-line treatments for this and many other conditions are conservative. It's also important to note that in pain medicine, complementary therapies such as massage and acupuncture are often very helpful.

Eliminating all pain is not always a realistic goal.

Many people wrongly assume that in this day and age with all of the different types of pain treatment—including opiate medications, which are typically reserved for postoperative and cancer pain as well as sometimes being used for other types of severe and refractory physical discomfort—that all pain can be relieved. This is simply not true. Pain is almost always a part of the healing process and while alleviating physical discomfort as much as possible is important, it's usually not possible to make this a completely painless journey. There are many reasons for this, but the most important one is that pain treatments can have serious side effects that make the risks outweigh the benefits. What this means is that while it is usually very safe to alleviate some discomfort, trying to get rid of all pain can mean the treatments are too aggressive and the risk of serious side effects too great. For example, opiate (narcotic) medications are usually safe to take, but even in small doses they may affect one's ability to think clearly and to react to different situations (which is why it is recommended that people don't take them and drive). In very high doses, they can impair breathing. In medicine, we call this the "risk-benefit profile" of a given treatment. The benefit of any given therapy needs to far outweigh the risk of serious side effects.

Alleviating pain is an important factor in healing, and though not all pain can easily or safely be relieved, reducing discomfort will help you to function better. Therefore, pay particular attention to this symptom and focus on strategies that will help alleviate your discomfort. Remember that when it comes to physical discomfort, toughing it out is not always the best strategy.

Healing Strategies

To help relieve pain, consider trying one or more of these strategies:

Analyze Your Pain

Think about where the pain is coming from, what is causing it, what makes it better, and what makes it worse. Then ask yourself what I always ask my patients, "What do you think will help?" My patients give me the answer all the time, because they know their bodies. However, some of them don't take the time to analyze their pain—often because they think they need to "just live with it."

Take Your Pain Medicine Before You Really Need It

If you take medicine for pain, try taking it earlier in the day, before the pain becomes very bothersome. I call this "staying ahead" of the pain symptoms. All medications for pain work better when it's not as severe. This is also true for the "next dose"—it will work better if you take it before the pain becomes really pronounced. Many of my patients try either ibuprofen or acetaminophen, medications that can be purchased without a prescription. When they tell me that these drugs don't work, I ask whether they've tried taking them earlier in the day. Sometimes, this simple solution works.

Try Complementary or Integrative Medicine Therapies

Complementary and alternative medicine, often abbreviated CAM, consists of many interventions that might be helpful to people. When these interventions have been studied and have some proven efficacy they are often called "integrative" therapies. Some of the therapies that you may want to explore include massage, acupuncture, progressive muscle relaxation, Reiki, meditation, and biofeedback.

Exercise Your Body

Exercise may help to alleviate pain; strong muscles help support your whole body. However, try to avoid activities that exacerbate the painful part of the body.

Apply a Hot or Cold Pack

Using a cold pack will do two important things—reduce inflammation and provide an anesthetic effect—whereas heat tends to relax the muscles. Think about what you may need to relieve your pain: Is it muscle relaxation or a reduction in inflammation and a numbing effect that you are after? You can also try alternating heat and cold. It's important to avoid both hot and cold burns. Use heat or cold for no more than twenty to thirty minutes at a time. Avoid packs that are too hot and don't use cold packs over areas that have poor blood supply (for example, if you have peripheral vascular disease it's best not to use a cold pack on your lower leg or foot).

Get Some Sleep

Remember that pain and sleep problems often go hand in hand. If you are having trouble sleeping, the forthcoming chapter on sleep (chapter 11) may help you.

Table 7.1 Commonly Used Pain Medications and Their Potential Side Effects*

Medication	Potential Side Effects
Acetaminophen	liver damage
Antidepressants	sedation, dry mouth, constipation, inability to urinate, weight gain
Antiseizure drugs	dizziness, nausea, blood or liver injury, sedation, weight gain
Lidocaine patch	skin irritation or rash
Muscle relaxants	dizziness, sedation, constipation, blood or liver injury
NSAIDs (nonsteroidal anti-inflammatory drugs)	gastrointestinal bleeding, injury to the kidneys, increased blood pressure
Opiates (narcotics)	rash/itching, nausea/vomiting, constipation, sedation, dizziness, cognitive impairment, difficulty breathing, urinary retention
Tramadol hydrochloride	nausea, vomiting, dry mouth, dizziness, sedation

*This is not a complete list of side effects.

Table 7.2 Nonpharmacologic Treatment for Pain

Acupuncture

Assistive devices (for example, a cane can help with a painful
    hip or knee)

Biofeedback

Braces or splints

Ergonomic equipment (for example, a telephone ear set can
    help with neck pain)

Exercise

Footwear/orthotics

Guided imagery

Hypnosis

Massage

Meditation

Modalities such as hot and cold packs

Relaxation therapy/stress reduction

Transcutaneous electrical nerve stimulation (TENS)

Ultrasound

Heal Yourself from the Outside In

chapter 8

You Can Benefit From the Love
of Others to Heal

I know a couple, now in their eighties, who I'll call Francine and George. Francine was born the daughter of Boston gentry in 1924. She was a debutante who met her husband, George, when she was eighteen years old. He must have been a dashing young man, because he's still handsome as an octogenarian. George was just a little more than one year older than Francine and became immediately smitten with the charming beauty. They married less than two years after they met. Shortly after they were married, Francine became pregnant and George went off to war to fly Piper Cubs over Germany. By the time he came home, there was a gorgeous fifteen-month-old daughter waiting for him.

The next few years were busy as George caught up on the time he missed with his wife and child, and went to business school. Francine became pregnant with their second child, but tragically she contracted a severe case of polio. Fortunately, after many months Francine recovered most of her strength and only in later years would her limp become noticeable when she was tired. Despite the war and polio, they were happy and George became a highly successful businessman. Francine stayed home and raised their children, and then in later years returned to her passion: art.

I've known Francine and George since they were in their sixties. I've always been impressed by their commitment to and enduring love for one another. They are partners, but have different interests. Francine is currently a well-respected artist whose work hangs in Boston's Museum of Fine Arts, and George is now a well-known Boston philanthropist. They are a striking couple; when I see them I think of the word "regal." As I've come to know them, there are many other words to describe these two people including devoted, caring, intelligent, and remarkable.

I asked Francine if she would share her story; it's truly an epic love story. She agreed, and told me that getting through the war, polio, breast cancer (hers), and prostate cancer (his), as well as raising three children and having successful careers was truly a team effort. They've been married well over six decades and Francine breaks those years down into three categories. The first she calls "Mad Love," which were the years filled with passion and physical love. The second she labels "Raising Your Children," which she says were years of joy. The third she says is "Huge Companionship." She is quick to say that the three categories overlap and there is still passion that withstands the passing of time.

When I asked her to look back and tell me what she knows in her eighties that she didn't know in her twenties she said, "I didn't know how subtly things would change." I also wondered whether she thought that her strong and enduring love for her husband helped her to heal from serious illnesses and to live a long life. She replied, "The support and the knowledge that you have someone solidly behind you helps immeasurably." Importantly, Francine emphasizes the cycle of life, and about the three children that she and George brought into this world, she says, "The companionship of your children as you get older is very precious."

How Our Relationships Affect Our Health

Connections to friends, loved ones, the community, and the environment are known to cause physical changes within the body that improves health and can help with physical healing. For example, some scientists hypothesize that levels of oxytocin, a hormone produced by the hypothalamus in the brain, is increased during positive social interactions. Oxytocin is probably best known for its important role in helping mothers and babies bond during breast-feeding. Oxytocin's role in other relationships is not well understood, but higher levels during positive social engagements may result in health benefits. Other hormones and biological compounds in our bodies likely play a role in the relationship between affection and wellness.

Psychiatrist Edward Hallowell believes that connections have such an important impact on health that he wrote a fascinating book on this topic. In *Connect,* Dr. Hallowell writes, "Connection is an essential vitamin. You can't live without it."

Indeed, the scientific evidence is overwhelming that our relationships have a powerful influence on our health. One rather clever study that was published in the *Journal of the American Medical Association* tested social ties and the susceptibility to the common cold. In this study, researchers placed drops of two different viruses into the noses of healthy volunteers. Taking into account a variety of factors including age, sex, weight, and so on, the conclusion was that people with more social ties were much less likely to become sick.

Many of the studies on health and relationships have been done with married couples. This research has demonstrated that good marriages tend to have a positive impact on survival, even in people who are critically ill. For example, in a study of more than ten thousand Israeli men, researchers found that a wife's love and support were important factors in reducing the risk of developing angina pectoris—a painful condition of the coronary arteries that results in decreased blood flow to the heart.

A study published in the *American Journal of Cardiology* found that "marital quality" improved survival in men and women with heart failure over a four-year study period. These researchers later published an eight-year follow-up study in 2006 that revealed that marital quality continued to predict survival—particularly in women.

If good relationships promote health and well-being, do strained relationships contribute to illness? The short answer is: yes. Although it's difficult to overgeneralize and say that all tense relationships cause or promote illness, many research studies support the hypothesis that toxic relationships are harmful to emotional and physical health. For example, one longitudinal study that was started in 1971 included participants of the Framingham Offspring Study, consisting of the children (and their spouses) of the original participants of the famous Framingham Heart Study. In the offspring study, Elaine Eaker, ScD, and colleagues evaluated nearly four thousand participants and found that marital conflict and strain were associated with adverse health outcomes. Of particular interest, the researchers reported that "self-silencing," defined as the tendency to keep your thoughts to yourself to avoid conflict in a relationship (repressed anger), led to decreased survival in women but not men.

Marital stress certainly may affect people physically. A study published in *Psychosomatic Medicine* examined how reactive couples' hearts were when they were exposed to marital stress. In this study, researchers recruited sixty couples whose average age was twenty-five years and who had been married an average of three years. Each couple was paid thirty dollars to participate, and they were told that the purpose of the study was to examine the cardiovascular effects of conversation. The couples were given topics to discuss and told to present either the same (agreement) or opposing (disagreement) sides of current event issues. Blood pressure and heart rate measurements were recorded during the interactions. The husbands' hostility scores correlated with greater rises in blood pressure, particularly when they tried to assert dominance in the interaction. Wives who disagreed with hostile husbands showed greater heart rate reactivity. Of course, these were young, healthy couples and one can only surmise the havoc that decades of stress on the heart can do to discordant partners.

Though many studies have been done evaluating the heart, this is not the only part of one's body that might be affected by strained relationships. During the 1990s, Janice Kiecolt-Glaser, Ph.D., and her husband, Ronald Glaser, Ph.D., and colleagues from Ohio State University published a series of provocative reports on how hostile marital interactions affect couples' immune systems and hormones. In one experiment titled "Negative Behavior During Marital Conflict is Associated with Immunological Down-Regulation," ninety newlywed couples were hospitalized for twenty-four hours and studied. Couples who exhibited more negative or hostile behaviors during a thirty-minute discussion of marital problems subsequently had a significant decrease in their immune function as tested by four immunological assays (blood tests) including diminished natural killer cell activity that is responsible for "immune surveillance" and helps to ward off infections and cancer. Another study by the same group of scientists evaluated older couples (mean age was sixty-seven years) who had been married an average of forty-two years. In this study an escalation of negative behavior during conflict and poor marital satisfaction revealed strong relationships to endocrine changes (hormones that the body produces, which are influenced by stress) including cortisol, adrenocorticotropic hormone (ACTH), and norepinephrine. The researchers concluded, "Abrasive marital interactions may have physiological consequences even among older adults in long-term marriages."

Another avenue of evaluating the impact of stressful relationships on health is how well experimentally induced wounds heal. In one study, investigators enrolled twenty-eight healthy women aged twenty-one to forty-five who were either in the process of a marital separation or were recently divorced (less than six months before). These women reported that they were very stressed and were compared to an age-matched control group of twenty-seven "happy" women. All of the women underwent a testing procedure on their cheeks. The skin test sites were disrupted by a non-painful method using sticky tape that removed layers of cells. Damage to the skin barrier was calculated using a tool and a mathematical equation that calculates an increase in water loss. The strength of the skin as a barrier was determined by how many tape strippings were required to disrupt the skin barrier. The researchers determined there was no difference between the two groups of women in this part of the experiment (that is, both groups of women had the same skin strength). Twenty-four hours later, most of the happy women had totally healed while several of the stressed women did not. This study showed that wound recovery was impaired by stress.

In a remarkable study published in the *Archives of General Psychiatry,* researchers evaluated how well couples with wounds healed. Each couple was admitted two times to a hospital research unit. During each admission, the participants were "wounded" with a skin-blistering technique. The researchers recorded how fast their wounds healed and how well the participants were able to produce levels of certain healing compounds (cytokines). The couples' relationships were studied and rated by researchers as "high hostile" or "low hostile." During the first admission, the couples were encouraged to have a positive interaction with each other and during the second admission, there was a conflict resolution task that produced a more negative interaction. Perhaps not surprisingly, high-hostile couples had significantly slower wound healing—their wounds healed at 60 percent of the rate of low-hostile couples. Comparing the two hospital admissions, both groups had slowed rates of wound healing during the second admission when stress was higher because the focus was on conflict resolution, but the low-hostile couples still healed faster.

Based on the results of many studies looking at physical healing and relationships, we know that love and support will help you recover and discord will slow your healing. As the authors of this study noted:

> Marriage is the central relationship for the majority of adults, and morbidity and mortality are reliably lower for married individuals than unmarried individuals across such diverse health threats as cancer, heart attacks, and surgery . . . the simple presence of a spouse is not necessarily protective; a troubled marriage is itself a prime source of stress, while simultaneously limiting the partner's ability to seek support in other relationships.

Though much of the research has been conducted with married couples, it is reasonable to say that it is the relationship, not the marriage certificate (or lack thereof) that influences people's health.

How Illness Affects Relationships

There is no doubt that illness has an effect on relationships. For some, the effect may be very positive. There are many stories of families reuniting after a loved one becomes ill. One woman I met told me that her bout with ovarian cancer was the clichéd "blessing in disguise" because it brought her estranged adult daughter back into the family fold.

However, while some relationships will easily endure and even strengthen during a medical crisis, others may suffer. Those of us who have experienced health problems are well aware that its impact is far-reaching. Friends and loved ones cannot and do not perfectly meet the challenge in every instance. Even a very committed loved one or a really good friend may experience "empathy fatigue." Illness and injury add considerable stress to our lives and often strain relationships.

A woman I'll call Lisa underwent breast cancer treatment several years ago. Lisa has an excellent prognosis and is doing well in all facets of her life with the exception of resuming physical intimacy with her husband. Despite her ability to resume most of the things that she used to enjoy, Lisa says that she is worried about having sex with her husband because she doesn't feel attractive. During her treatment she had surgery, which left a small scar on her breast, and chemotherapy, in which she lost her hair and gained some weight. Though her hair has returned, she is still self-conscious about the scar on her breast and her weight gain. She makes no overtures to her husband because she doesn't want to "lead him on."

On the other hand, many couples resume a loving and physically intimate relationship right away. Journalist and producer Geralyn Lucas wrote about how she and her husband had sex almost immediately following her mastectomy for breast cancer. Though at first she wasn't sure how her husband would react sexually, he led the way and she reciprocated. Geralyn shared this experience and how it helped her realize the depth of her husband's love for her. She wrote:

> I put on some perfume. And I line my lips with lipstick. I can't even feel Tyler's hand when he puts it on the bright red diagonal scar across my chest. In fact, I have been walking into strangers with my reconstructed right boob because I cannot feel where it starts.
>
> But the great thing about sex is that it's like riding a bicycle. I know that Tyler still loves me—my laugh, our conversations—but will he still be turned on?
>
> Yes, yes, and definitely yes. I cannot believe that Tyler wants me so much.
>
> The way he is kissing me and touching me, I know that it's not my hair or my boob that ever made him fall in love with me. It was my mojo. It was always there, just waiting for me to meet it.

After Tyler and I have sex again I feel so hot that I still can't get that Shania Twain song out of my head: *Man, I feel like a woman!*

Geralyn and I met when we were in a New York City television studio's "green room," waiting to be interviewed. When I told her I was going to use this passage in a book I was writing, she laughed and said that it was all true.

Giving and Receiving Love

Relationships, of course, require the participation of two people. Thus, there is a natural giving and receiving of affection and practical support. Usually, the more committed each person is to the nurturing of the other, the better the union. Still, many relationships are unbalanced with one person doing most of the nurturing, which is not always problematic or unnatural. An obvious example is a parent-child bond. However, in liaisons where partners should be equal in their affection and support of each other, sometimes one person does more of the "giving."

It's normal for relationships to have an ebb and flow to them, in which the amount of nurturing needed and provided depends on many factors. Serious illness is certainly a time when changes may occur in how someone gives and receives love. During my treatment for cancer, I experienced an outpouring of love from my friends and colleagues. Perfect for healing, right? Well, yes and no. I very much appreciated their devotion and kindness, but sometimes it was hard to accept. For instance, I had always been the parent in charge of cooking my children's meals. When I was ill, friends cooked for us. I was grateful for their assistance, while at the same time I wanted to be the one who cared for my children's needs.

For some people, illness can wreak havoc with relationships. Two cornerstones of serious illness, dependency and suffering, can certainly shake the foundations of even the strongest bonds. Psychologist Harriet Lerner reminds us, though, that this is a necessary and important aspect of the human condition. In her book *The Dance of Connection,* she tells readers, "Dependency and suffering are essential components of the human condition. Sooner or later harsh experience teaches us how much we need each other. The only aspect of either that's really shameful is the persistent and false societal belief that people can bootstrap their way to health, wealth, and happiness."

Nevertheless, serious medical problems can, and often do, marginalize one's role in a relationship. A parent may become less essential to her children as they begin to rely on others. Or, an adolescent may become increasingly reliant on a parent, thus impacting the normal transition into adulthood. I recall one of my good friends in high school telling me about how upset he was when, after breaking both of his arms in a car accident, he needed to rely on his mother to help him go to the bathroom. As high school kids sometimes do, he described this in graphic detail. I understood, even as a teenager, that as he was transitioning into manhood, having his mother be responsible for wiping his bottom, much as she did when he was a baby, was extremely difficult for him. All relationships are subject to change, albeit perhaps only temporarily, when one person is in the process of healing.

The challenge during this time is to be able to graciously accept the love and nurturing that others bestow upon you while at the same time continuing to try to nurture them in return.

When People Aren't Paying Attention, Don't Assume They Don't Care

There are many medical crises that instantly bring people together. For example, when someone is seriously injured in a car accident or is diagnosed with cancer, friends and loved ones usually band together to provide emotional and practical support. However, there are many other serious medical conditions that don't bring about the same level of empathy and aid. This subdued response from friends and family members is almost always due to a lack of understanding about the diagnosis, symptoms, and what the individual might need in terms of support.

For instance, a young woman with multiple sclerosis may appear healthy to others but may be struggling physically due to weakness with walking and daily activities such as taking care of her home or going to work where she has to climb stairs or walk through long corridors to get to her office. Though she may wish that others were more attentive to her struggle, friends and family view her as self-sufficient and not in need of either emotional or practical support. Even in a crisis-type diagnosis, such as cancer, loved ones may provide support up to a certain point and then with-draw when they view the crisis as being over. For those di-agnosed with cancer, this retreat often begins when the individual is at his lowest point physically—at the end of chemotherapy or other treatments.

Everyone can benefit from emotional support and many will also be helped by practical support. Even if you can be completely independent and you don't need to rely on oth-ers for practical support, now might be a good time to ac-cept help as it is best to use the energy you have to recover as well as you possibly can. For instance, if you are able to go grocery shopping, but it leaves you too tired to exercise, that is not a good trade-off. The exercise is more important to someone who is in need of healing. Tasks that serve to wear you out rather than help you recover should be dele-gated whenever possible.

Engaging friends and loved ones is often as simple as sharing with them more about what you are currently going through. Confiding in people you trust frequently leads to them inquiring as to how they can help. If they do, give them specific answers so that their assistance is truly useful. If they don't offer to help, consider asking them outright. Most people truly find it a source of joy to help others, as you probably do. However, while it is taking a bit of a risk to ask someone for support, keep in mind that they might be worried about being rebuffed if they offer assistance. Though some people may not jump at the chance to help, most people who are not forthcoming are simply waiting for you to take the initiative and let them know what is the best way to nurture you during this time.

Some people may feel that they are relying too heavily or even "using" their friends or other loved ones to help them when they are healing. Using people suggests that one is being disingenuous and perhaps even dishonest. Surrounding yourself with people who nurture and support you, and who in turn you nurture and support, is an integral part not only of healing well, but living a worthwhile life. Also, just as they are helping you to recover so too are you (by letting them nurture and gracefully receiving their help and affection) contributing to their health.

There is no doubt that making new connections can be hard when you are ill. In her memoir, Joni Rodgers, a young woman diagnosed with non-Hodgkin's lymphoma, recited a pretend conversation that she might have with a new acquaintance: "Hi, I'm Joni, and I'm a sucking black hole of emotional need right now. My hobbies are taking drugs, napping, and calling people I hardly know for emergency child-care. Wanna be my friend?" I like this fictitious conversation because it's clever, but also because it resonates with how I felt when I was undergoing treatment for cancer. I am normally an outgoing person who likes to meet new people. But when I was ill, I felt vulnerable and was much less open to connecting with others—especially if I didn't know them very well.

You may want to focus on making new connections, but if you feel vulnerable (as I did), you can work on connections you already have. This might be calling an old friend you have lost touch with or writing a loving letter to your partner or one of your children. Most of us have many people we can connect with but are often too busy or too distracted to do so. Pausing for a few minutes to chat with people you come into contact with can help you to feel much more connected. These brief interactions may lead to deeper bonds as over time you learn the names and stories of these individuals.

While you work on strengthening your connections, one trap to avoid is to overly rely on the Internet. The Internet is often thought of as the ultimate in connections because of its speed and far reaching capacity. But, the Internet can actually *decrease* your social capital. In a study titled "Internet Paradox," researchers examined the effects of the Internet on social involvement and psychological well being in more than 150 people during their first one to two years online. They found that participants overall used the Internet quite extensively for communication. "Nonetheless," the scientists wrote, "greater use of the Internet was associated with declines in participants' communication with family members in the household, declines in the size of their social circle, and increases in their depression and loneliness."

If you have a close relationship with someone that is not going well, you may want to consider separating yourself a bit from that person. However, this might not be desirable or feasible if the person you are in conflict with is your partner or a family member.

Love, social capital (this term is used to define all of your social relationships and connections; those who are "rich" in social capital benefit significantly in terms of their health), and all of the connections that surround you, can facilitate your ability to mend. Physician Oliver Wendell Holmes once said, "The sound of a kiss is not so loud as that of a cannon, but its echo lasts a great deal longer." Illness may create problems in your relationships and may contribute to feeling lonely and isolated. Consciously counteracting that tendency is important and will help you to heal. Dr. Hallowell summed it up quite elegantly when he wrote, "Life is loss . . . To oppose the pain of loss, we use a human glue, the force of love. The force of love creates our many different connections. This is what saves us all."

Healing Strategies

Strengthening Your Relationships and Building Social Capital

1. Reestablish contact with an old friend.
2. Write a love letter to each of your children and/or your partner.
3. Join a support group and attend the meetings.
4. Plan a weekly date with a friend (it doesn't have to be the same person every week).

5. Meet a friend for a walk at least once a week.

6. Warmly greet people who you see but don't really know (for example, the mailman or check-out person in the grocery store). Learn their names and a bit about them.

7. Sign up for a class (yoga, woodworking, journal writing, or the like).

8. Attend an event in your community (pancake breakfast, school concert, town meeting, bingo, and so on).

9. Sign up to participate in an event that supports a charitable cause (such as a walkathon or a crafts fair).

10. Volunteer one morning or afternoon a week in your community (perhaps at your school library, local hospital, or senior center).

11. Resume or increase intimacy with your partner at regular intervals at a level that is satisfying for both of you.

chapter 9

You Can Eat to Heal

There is no doubt that what you eat can help you to heal. For example, vitamin D has so much research to support its powerful effect on our immune systems and healing that I often call it vitamin D-ivine. Vitamin A is necessary for skin and bones to heal well and has a role in immune function. Vitamin C is necessary for collagen formation and optimal immune function, and it works as a tissue antioxidant. Vitamin E is a potent antioxidant. Bromelain (a group of enzymes that are derived from the pineapple plant) reduces swelling, bruising, and pain, and improves healing time following trauma or surgery. Glucosamine is an important factor in wound healing. Adequate protein is absolutely essential for optimal healing and specific amino acids, the building blocks of protein, that seem to play a significant role include arginine and glutamine. Zinc is required for DNA synthesis, cell growth, and protein synthesis. This is a short and incomplete list. However, the point here is that food provides many, many incredibly important substances that assist with healing.

It would be interesting but unethical to conduct a study on people who were in need of healing and divide them into two groups—one that receives a nutritious diet and the other group that does not. However, an interesting study that was done looked at healthy national level judo athletes. In this study, one group underwent a significant food restriction while the other group (the control group) didn't. The purpose of this research was to determine whether food restriction affected physical performance and levels of certain compounds in the body. At the end of the study, all of the men reported to a gymnastic hall where they had the same breakfast, weighed in, had blood samples taken, and performed some other tests such as a grip strength measurement. They then had a simulated judo competition.

The results were quite remarkable though not surprising. In the dietary restricted group, the blood chemistries were significantly altered (for example, there was a decrease in testosterone and insulin, and an increase in cortisol and other compounds). Physical performance was also significantly affected, with the dietary restricted group performing poorly on grip strength and horizontal rowing tests. This group also reported a decrease in "vigor" and an increase in fatigue and tension. The authors of this study concluded that poor and restricted nutrition "affects the physiology and psychology of judo athletes and impairs physical performance." Though I doubt there will be studies done like this on people who are ill or injured, the foregone conclusion is that diet will have a major impact. In fact, it's reasonable to hypothesize that nutrition will have a far greater impact on those who are in need of healing than in supremely conditioned athletes.

The easiest and best way to ensure that your body gets the many ingredients that will help it to heal effectively is to eat a nutritious and varied diet. Taking a lot of supplements is not usually a good idea for a number of reasons, including that you may be taking a dose that is excessive. The supplement may contain other ingredients that are harmful, or it may be missing ingredients that food contains that help a particular substance work ideally. Additionally the supplement may interact with your prescription medications rendering them less effective (St. John's wort is a good example of a supplement that interacts with many prescription drugs).

I am always fascinated by the concept of "if a little is good, then more is better." While this may apply to money, it definitely does not work well with what you put in your body. Nevertheless, many people either consciously or unwittingly take megadoses of vitamins and others supplements, erroneously believing it is good for them. For example, one of my former patients is a Catholic nun who has taken a vow of poverty. What little money she has she spends on supplements. One day she brought in a shopping bag full of what she takes on a daily basis. I examined the various pills and showed her that she was taking much more than 100 percent of the recommended daily allowance (RDA). In fact, for several vitamins she was consuming as much as 5,000 percent of the RDA. Multiply that by 365 days per year and she is consuming just under two million times the RDA. It's hard to imagine a scenario where someone would need nearly two million extra doses of a vitamin in a given year. Moreover, it's much more likely (and this is borne out by the research studies) that megadosing can have some very harmful health effects.

When I pointed this out to my patient, she instantly recognized that she was taking a huge amount of unnecessary and potentially harmful supplements. However, being the frugal woman that she is, she told me that while she wouldn't buy any more supplements, she was going to finish what she had so that the money she had spent on them "wouldn't go to waste."

Megadosing isn't the only problem with supplements. Even if you take a reasonable amount of a given product, there still is the potential for serious side effects. For example, a study performed by Dr. Robert Saper and colleagues at Harvard Medical School that was published in the highly respected *Journal of the American Medical Association,* found that there was a significant and potentially quite toxic level of heavy metal content in ayurvedic herbal medicine products. The results from this study are as follows:

> Lead, mercury, and arsenic intoxication have been associated with the use of Ayurvedic herbal medicine products . . . One of 5 Ayurvedic herbal medicine products produced in South Asia and available in Boston South Asian grocery stores contains potentially harmful levels of lead, mercury, and/or arsenic. Users of Ayurvedic medicine may be at risk for heavy metal tox-

icity, and testing of Ayurvedic herbal medicine products for toxic heavy metals should be mandatory.

Supplements, whether they are in the form of vitamins, ayurvedic products, or other substances, are not regulated and may contain ingredients that are not good for you. Some people think that because they purchase a product in a health food store, that product is safe and will make them healthier. This is not true and it's important to use all supplements cautiously.

This goes back to my main point, which is that *the best way to get the ingredients you need to heal well is by eating a nutritious and varied diet.* The one supplement that I do routinely recommend to people is a single multivitamin that acts as an "insurance policy" to ensure that you get enough of the essential vitamins in your diet.

I am definitely not opposed to using supplements in general. It is the *misuse* and *overuse* of supplements that I caution against. There are many supplements that doctors will recommend based on the scientific literature supporting their use. For example, one study evaluating the use of fish oil (omega-3 fatty acids) combined with olive oil showed a significant improvement in joint pain, morning stiffness, and grip strength in people with rheumatoid arthritis. Another study showed that fish oil supplements may confer some benefit in patients with multiple sclerosis. I recommend supplements to some of my patients in very specific cases (for example, additional calcium and vitamin D are usually a good idea), but before you take additional supplements, I suggest you talk to your doctor about whether they are necessary and what are the potential risks and benefits of taking them.

Before I leave the topic of megadosing, I want to mention that supplements are not the only way this may occur. For example, foods and beverages that are fortified with vitamins and minerals may pose a problem if the doses are too high. Some of these products are being marketed as "functional foods" and are promoted as being healthier for people because they are fortified. However, again, too much of a good thing is not always wise, so keep this in mind when you eat.

Healing Strategies

There is no single perfect diet that we know of at this time, and it's hard to imagine with different ethnic backgrounds, geographic locales, and individual food preferences, that there will ever be a single "perfect diet." Instead, the best diet will likely always be one that is obtained by eating a variety of nutritious foods. Of course, this advice is too general to be very helpful; nevertheless, no matter what you like to eat, you can use food to help you heal if you implement some or all of these eight strategies.

1. Eat three small to medium meals each day with two healthy snacks.
2. Be sure to get enough protein and complex carbohydrates in your diet.

3. Eat five or more servings of colorful fruits and vegetables daily.
4. If you need to gain or lose weight, talk to your doctor and a nutritionist or registered dietician.
5. Take a daily multivitamin and get enough calcium and vitamin D.
6. Drink plenty of water.
7. Try to eat certified organic foods whenever possible.
8. Avoid nicotine completely and alcohol as much as possible.

More About the Eight Strategies

1. Eat three small to medium meals each day with two healthy snacks.

One of the main complaints that people have after a serious injury or illness is profound fatigue. This fatigue can be due to many factors that are covered in greater detail in the next chapter. However, one important consideration in treating fatigue is to look at the role that food plays in energy. Food, of course, is our body's fuel. Keeping our tank full without overindulging is important. Think of driving your car, how often do you let your gas tank get to empty and then run out of fuel in the middle of your ride? If you are like most people, you either never do that or very rarely. Instead, you keep a bit of gas in the tank at all times, so you never run out. It works well to fuel your body in this way as well. It's not ideal to have big spikes in blood sugar levels followed a short time later by big drops with an energy "bottoming out" effect. Instead, if you can eat to fuel your body so that you have a consistent and stable level of energy, you'll feel and heal better. If you have any special dietary concerns, including diabetes, you should check with your doctor before trying this.

2. Be sure to get enough protein and complex carbohydrates in your diet.

Both protein and carbohydrates are good energy sources for our bodies. Carbohydrates are more readily available to be used as energy, so it's important not to eliminate them from your diet. Carbohydrates can be classified as "complex" (vegetables, nuts, seeds, legumes, and whole grains) and "simple" (bread, pasta, and other starches). Sometimes, a third class is mentioned that contains "sugars" (table sugar, honey, and sweets such as candy). All carbohydrates are broken down into sugar when digested. This sugar enters the bloodstream and the pancreas responds by releasing insulin to lower the "blood sugar" level. This process is often referred to as a glycemic index—which is a method of measuring how fast and how high a person's blood sugar level rises. *You want to eat foods that have a low glycemic level because these don't cause such fast and high fluctuations in blood sugar levels.* Complex carbohydrates fulfill this goal.

Complex carbohydrate sources (listed in Table 9.1) include whole grains, which differ from refined grains in that they contain the germ (sprout of a new plant), endosperm (the seed's source of energy), and bran (the outer layer). Refined grains (such as white flour) have the bran and germ, which contain important nutrients, removed during the milling process. Some of the nutrients that may be lost include B vitamins, iron, zinc, phytochemicals, vitamin E, and fiber. Moreover, milling the grain means that it is digested more quickly and therefore causes a faster and higher blood sugar level. Your body reacts to the raised blood sugar levels by releasing a large amount of insulin from the pancreas to lower the level, which in turn causes a precipitous drop in blood sugar level. This is exactly what you don't want when you are trying to heal well. Instead, you want a consistent and comfortable blood sugar level rather than large spikes followed by dips.

Protein is used as energy but also helps cells recover and regenerate. In some types of serious illness, such as extensive burns or during chemotherapy, there is an increased need for protein to help with cellular recovery. Generally, it's a good idea to get about 15 percent to 20 percent of your calories from protein. For people healing from a serious injury or illness, I usually recommend they aim for the higher end of this range and sometimes even go beyond that. If your body has undergone extensive cellular injury, it's a good idea to talk to your doctor and to meet with a registered dietician about what your specific protein needs might be. There are ways to measure someone's current protein status and needs, and this is very helpful in cases where there is a lot of cell injury.

In terms of protein sources, plant-based proteins (such as beans and nuts) have some advantages over animal proteins. Plant-based proteins provide phytochemicals (which can help with healing), vitamins, minerals, "good" fats, and fiber (fiber is found only in plant food). Table 9.2 provides a list of sources of vegetarian protein (I include dairy in this category).

3. *Eat five or more servings of colorful fruits and vegetables daily.*

Fruits and vegetables are quite remarkable for their many healing components. These foods are rich in vitamins, minerals, and other substances (such as phytochemicals) that can promote physical recovery. Eating at least five servings each day of fruits and vegetables is one of the best things you can do for your body. For example, the oft-touted healing properties of vitamin C are well deserved. Vitamin C helps with healing wounds and a deficiency leads to delayed wound healing and an increase in blood vessel (capillary) fragility as well as a reduced ability to ward off infection. Megadoses of vitamin C (such as the 18,000 milligrams proposed by scientist Linus Pauling as the daily dose) are not believed to be helpful and might in fact be harmful. While vitamin C deficiency slows healing, high doses (greater than 2,000 milligrams per day) have not been shown to accelerate healing. If you eat a diet rich in fruits and vegetables, you will get plenty of vitamin C and other vitamins that help with healing.

Fruits and vegetables are also good sources of antioxidants—a subcategory of phytochemicals. Diets high in antioxidants are believed to help with healing. Antioxidants such as vitamins C and E, beta-carotene, and lycopene are found in many foods in this category. Lycopene is believed to be a particularly powerful antioxidant, and is found in tomatoes, apricots, guava, watermelon, papaya, and pink grapefruit. As a general rule, it is helpful to remember that darkly colored fruits and vegetables are richer in phyto-chemicals and antioxidants.

There are other substances, some of which we have iden-tified and some of which are still unknown, that are present in these foods and help with healing. These include carot-enoids (orange colored foods including carrots, yams, apri-cots, and cantaloupe), anthocyanins (tomatoes, red peppers, and red grapefruit juice), and sulfides (garlic and onions).

In some studies, fruit and vegetable supplements that come in pill form have been shown to raise antioxidant lev-els in the blood. The primary concern with these supple-ments is that while we know that fruits and vegetables are extremely important in helping to prevent certain kinds of cancer, we aren't precisely sure which ingredients are the most important. Moreover, there are likely things in these foods that we haven't even identified yet. What this means is that fruit and vegetable supplements, while they might be helpful, are almost certainly not as good as eating your daily five or more servings of these foods. I generally recommend a supplement for my patients only when it is clear that they are not consuming fruits and vegetables and are unable to change their diet to include at least some of these.

Taking nutritional supplements that contain megadoses of vitamins or antioxidants is not recommended. At present, the issue of taking supplements that contain antioxidants is a source of much debate in the medical community. While it is true that increasing the phytochemicals in your diet is an excellent idea, taking supplements might not be wise. There is some evidence to suggest that the old adage "too much of a good thing isn't so good" is applicable to antioxidants. The concept of "oxidative stress," which has not been fully explored, is thought to be an issue relating to taking too many antioxidants which might actually depress rather than enhance one's immune system.

Minerals, too, have their role in healing. For example, zinc is an essential mineral that helps with protein synthesis and wound healing. Zinc also plays a role in immune function. Zinc deficiency causes loss of appetite, impaired immune function, and delayed wound healing. Again, if you eat plenty of fruits and vegetables it is unlikely that you will need to take a zinc supplement; taking too much zinc (in a supplement form) can inhibit healing and may even cause a copper deficiency, which can also lead to impaired healing.

4. If you need to gain or lose weight, talk to your doctor and a nutritionist or registered dietician.

When you've been seriously ill, gaining or losing weight is something that is good to get some professional advice about. However, with any diet, it's important to consider the total number of calories and the fat content. Fat, along with protein and carbohydrates, is an energy source that your body needs to function well. Most people don't have to worry about needing more calories or fat in their diets. As a matter of fact, the current trend is that usually people eat an excess of calories and get too much fat in their diets. Therefore, I usually recommend that people stick with a low fat diet while they are healing, which helps with calorie control as well. However, there are instances when someone has lost a lot of weight and is in need of replenishing his or her fat stores. To do this, one may need to both increase the total number of calories and the dietary fat content. Trying to either lose or gain weight during your recovery is something that is important to discuss with your doctor and a registered dietician.

On average, people should eat about 10-15 calories for each pound they weigh in order to maintain their weight. If you want to gain weight, you'll need to eat additional calories (around 500 extra calories per day is a reasonable number to shoot for and will increase weight gain by about one pound per week). If you want to lose weight, you'll need to eat fewer calories. However, it is important to be sure and consume enough calories to keep up your energy level. If you don't eat enough calories, while you may lose weight more quickly, you'll feel lousy. If weight loss is a goal, do this gradually so that your energy level is optimal.

As you consider the fat in your diet, it's best to stick to small amounts of polyunsaturated and monounsaturated fats, which are considered "good fats." Saturated fats (for example, whole milk and high-fat meats) and trans fats (such as margarine, vegetable shortening, packaged breads, cakes, cookies, and crackers) are "bad fats" and it's a good idea to eat these in very limited quantities or to avoid them completely. Vegetable oils (such as grape seed, corn, olive, and canola), nuts, and some fish (such as salmon, lake trout, tuna, and herring) are sources of "good fats."

5. Take a daily multivitamin and get enough calcium and vitamin D.

Taking a multivitamin on a daily basis can help to ensure that you are getting what you need. Not everyone may need to take a multivitamin; however, most people can benefit from taking one as a sort of "insurance policy." For those who are anemic due to an iron deficiency this can be helpful as well. However, iron can contribute to constipation, so if you are not deficient in iron, and you are concerned about constipation, go with one of the low iron multivitamins (often labeled as a "senior" or geriatric alternative). Choose a multivitamin that does not exceed 100 percent of the U.S. recommended daily allowance (RDA); there is no difference between natural or synthetic brands.

Bone health is also very important, particularly if you have sustained injuries to your bones (for example, bone bruises or fractures), but also if you are not as active as you used to be. Many medications also have the side effect of decreasing bone density and making them more "brittle." When it comes to calcium and vitamin D supplements, these can vary quite a bit based on your age, sex, medical condition, and so on. Therefore, if you have concerns about your bones, talk to your doctor about this. Also, keep in mind that regular weight-bearing exercise helps to promote stronger bones (unless you have bone fractures that require a non- or partial-weight-bearing approach to healing) and that caffeine, alcohol, and tobacco can all have a negative impact on bone healing and bone density.

6. Drink plenty of water.

Water is the best way to hydrate your body and good hydration helps with healing. You need to take in fluid to have adequate blood circulating throughout your body transporting important healing substances to your cells and organs and carrying away waste materials. Dehydration can result in poor wound healing and other uncomfortable side effects such as constipation. Most people should drink six to eight glasses of water each day while they are trying to heal. If you have kidney problems or congestive heart failure, this might be too much. If you are on a very high protein diet, have draining wounds, are vomiting a lot, or have a chronic fever, this may be too little. Again, check with your doctor if you are not sure how much liquid you should be drinking.

7. Try to eat certified organic foods whenever possible.

We don't know very much about the long-term effects of the added chemicals that are commonly used to grow or preserve food. In the future, we will likely find out that such things as bovine growth hormone and irradiated or genetically engineered food are either not particularly harmful or that they can contribute to serious health problems. *It is unlikely that we'll find out that these things will be good for our health.* Therefore, when people ask me whether they should eat organic food, my answer is that it is wise to incorporate as much certified organic food as possible into your diet. Note well: only produce labeled as organic is certified as meeting USDA (United States Department of Agriculture) organic standards; "natural" does *not* mean organic.

Certified organic food, though sometimes more expensive than conventional food, is grown with a number of restrictions. For example, organic farmers in the meat industry don't give antibiotics or growth hormones to the animals. Organic food is also devoid of conventional pesticides, fertilizers, and ionizing radiation. The National Organic Program (NOP) is a federal law that requires all organic food products to meet the same standards and be certified under the same certification process. Along with this program, the USDA has developed strict labeling rules to help consumers know the specific content of the organic food they buy. The USDA Organic seal means that at least 95 percent of the product is organic.

If organic foods are not an option, then be sure to wash fruits and vegetables thoroughly under clean, cold running water before eating them. Wash thoroughly even if the produce will be cooked, peeled, or cut. Avoid using rinses, soaps, or chlorine bleach solutions.

8. Avoid nicotine completely and alcohol as much as possible.

Nicotine, especially in the form of cigarettes, is very toxic to healing tissues. Many studies have shown that smoking causes delays in wound healing and prevents optimal recovery. There are a number of well-studied reasons for this that were summarized in a review titled "Cutaneous Effects of Smoking." In this article in the *Journal of Cutaneous Medicine and Surgery*, the authors explained the technical reasons why nicotine inhibits healing, "Smoking has been shown to significantly decrease the immune response, leading to poor wound healing. In particular, smoking decreases interleukin-1 production, inhibits the early signals for B-cell transduction pathways, decreases cytotoxicity of natural killer cells, and causes T-cell anergy." What this boils down to is that smoking affects the immune system in a number of ways that can delay or inhibit healing. So, nicotine can act as a direct toxin that affects the immune system and it also can act indirectly to slow or impair healing by reducing blood flow to the injured area.

Most people begin smoking in their youth when they are the most vulnerable, the least knowledgeable, and years away from realizing the ill health effects of nicotine. When I talk to my patients about smoking, I always tread lightly. I know that they beat themselves up over this issue, and the last thing I want to do is to cause them more distress. I encourage my patients to view all previous attempts at stopping smoking as short-term successes—even if it was just for a day or two. This strategy of giving oneself credit for past short-term successes, whether the issue is smoking, weight loss, or anything else, is a powerful motivator and can lead to long-term success. Therefore, if you have tried to stop in the past and have been able to do so even for a short period of time, you have had some success at this. Moreover, this is probably a time in your life when you are extremely motivated to quit smoking. Increased motivation along with your past short-term successes, can be the keys to stopping forever.

Alcohol is a misunderstood and misrepresented substance that is definitely not helpful in healing from serious injury or illness. Though there is a small bit of inconclusive research that suggests alcohol in unknown but probably quite small quantities may be somewhat helpful in preventing heart disease, there is a much larger body of research that recognizes the very harmful effects of alcohol. Alcohol has been linked to a number of serious medical conditions including dementia, liver cirrhosis, and cancer. Since this is a book about physical healing, I will focus on how alcohol hinders this process.

One of the effects of alcohol is that it is toxic to nerves. Therefore, if you have an illness or injury that has compromised your nerve function, it's important not to add a nerve toxin to your body. In all likelihood, your nerves will heal better and more completely if you don't drink alcohol.

Alcohol also affects the immune system in a negative manner. Part of the reason for this likely has to do with alcohol's effect on cytokines, which are important chemicals produced by our bodies to help regulate healing and our immune systems. In a research article titled "Cytokines and Alcohol," the authors noted, "Alcohol use alters immune defenses against infections and results in increased incidence of bacterial pneumonias, a higher rate of chronic hepatitis C infections, and increases susceptibility to HIV infection." While these particular medical conditions may not concern you, it's important to recognize that alcohol travels throughout your body and may increase the damage to injured cells and organs if you are in need of healing for any reason.

Sometimes, people use alcohol for "medicinal reasons" to help control their mood or decrease their stress or improve their pain. Alcohol is not good medicine and may even have the opposite effect that one desires (for example, when used to improve one's mood, it often works as a depressant and makes someone feel worse). If you are using alcohol in a medicinal manner, talk to your doctor about strategies that would be more helpful.

Though alcohol won't help you to heal, it is important to note that an occasional drink or two is unlikely to do any harm. Alcohol seems to be the most detrimental when people either drink occasionally in excess or drink regularly, even in moderation. Therefore, if you drink in moderation for special occasions only, that will likely not affect your ability to heal well.

I often give motivational speeches on healing. I enjoy the challenge of speaking to impart an important message, while at the same time choosing language and stories that entertain. One occasion was at a big theater in Ohio; it was a lecture series that has been in existence for more than fifty years. The event coordinators told me, "Most of the people we invite to speak are really famous. You're not. So, you'll have to make sure that you offer the audience really meaningful information."

I only had forty minutes to speak, and the topic was on

how to heal optimally. Since diet is one of the three most important factors in healing, I spoke about some of the information that appears in this chapter. After the event there was a luncheon. One woman with pure white hair, sparkling eyes, and a bounce in her step came up to me and commented, "Dearie, I liked what you said, but I'm eighty-six years old and healthy. I'm going to keep taking all of my supplements, and I'm not going to follow any of your advice."

Rather than be offended, I always enjoy when people come up to me and (usually very politely) tell me things like this. The truth is that whether it's genes or diet or supplements or whatever, this woman is doing well and doesn't need to follow my advice. However, as I gently explained to this lovely lady, my recommendations are not geared for eighty-six-year-old healthy women. Instead, I offer advice for those who are in need of healing. If you are working toward better health, consider the information in this chapter, and most of all, pay attention to what you are putting into your body in order for it to heal optimally. At the same time, remember that the Bill Clinton "one step rule" does not apply to diet. You can't eat one wrong thing or even a bunch of junk food, and then anticipate disastrous results. Your body can handle quite a bit, and while paying attention to how you nourish it is important, worrying about every bite is not worthwhile or necessary.

Table 9.1 Sources of Complex Carbohydrates

Arborio rice

Barley rice

Basmati

Black, fava, kidney, lima, mung, navy, pinto, and white beans*

Bran

Brown and wild rice

Bulgur

Chickpeas

Flaxseeds

Fresh fruits

Fresh vegetables

Kasha

Millet

Oats

Rye

Whole grain wheat breads

Whole grain breakfast cereal (100 percent)

*Beans have the added benefit of being high in protein, too.

Table 9.2 Sources of Vegetarian Protein

Brown rice
Cottage cheese
Eggs
Legumes
Lentils
Meat analogs (such as "veggie burgers")
Nut and seed butters
Nuts
Quinoa
Quorn
Seeds
Soy milk
Tempeh
Tofu
Yogurt

Table 9.3 Sources of Vegetarian Iron

Blackstrap molasses
Beans
Bean sprouts
Bran
Cereal (some fortified cereals)
Dried fruit
Green leafy vegetables
Lentils
Parsley
Prune juice
Sesame seeds
Soybean nuts
Spinach
Yeast extract

Table 9.4 Sources of Vegetarian Vitamin B12

Alfalfa sprouts
Blue-green algae (spirulina, chlorella) and seaweeds
Dairy
Eggs
Milk
Miso
Soy milk (fortified)
Tamari
Tempeh
Yeast extract
Yogurt

Table 9.5 Eating to Improve Energy

- Be sure you are getting enough protein and complex carbohydrates in your diet.
- Don't skip any meals.
- Try eating three small to medium-size meals with two nutritious snacks in between.
- Avoid refined sugar and simple carbohydrates (such as sweets, crackers, and chips). These tend to give you a quick energy boost by increasing your blood sugar to a fairly high level which is followed by a precipitous drop—making you feel sluggish and tired.
- Take in adequate calories.
- If you are anemic (your doctor can tell you if you have anemia and the cause), you can increase your dietary intake of whatever you are deficient in (for example, iron or vitamin B12) to help improve this.
- Stay well hydrated. The best drinks are water, fruit and vegetable juices, and milk. It is best to avoid or limit your intake of caffeinated drinks (including coffees and teas), sodas, and alcohol.

chapter 10

You Can Use Exercise to Heal

If there was a chemical formula for exercise that could be packaged as a pill, there is no doubt it would be the most popular prescription drug available. Everyone knows that exercise helps keep people healthy, but how does it work to help us heal when we are seriously ill or injured?

Exercise helps many organs and tissues heal, such as muscles, bones, tendons, and ligaments. For example, the formation or *synthesis* of collagen helps injured tissues, such as tendons, to heal. Collagen gives structures in our body strength. You can think of collagen as the bricks that support many of our body's structures. Thus, collagen synthesis is very important in healing, especially after surgery or trauma. In a study that assessed how exercise affected the collagen at a muscle and tendon at the knee, researchers found that "there is a rapid increase in collagen synthesis after strenuous exercise in human tendon and muscle." Another factor is that exercise appears to decrease excessive scar tissue, called *fibrosis*. In one study, excessive scar tissue was diminished by 50 percent with exercise. These are examples of how exercise can help you to heal *better.*

While exercise is extremely important in helping us to recapture our former strength and vitality, it also helps us to actually heal *faster.* For example, in the study I just mentioned on scar tissue, the increase in collagen synthesis after exercise strongly suggests that exercise helps us to heal *better* and *faster.* In another experiment evaluating the benefits of exercise on wound healing, researchers assessed an initial group of twenty-eight sedentary older adults who were known to be in good health. It was hypothesized that a three-month program of aerobic exercise would significantly enhance wound healing. The participants were separated into two groups: a control group that didn't exercise and an exercise group. Each subject underwent a wound procedure that is a low-risk punch biopsy used in dermatological research. This 3.5 mm wound was placed on the back of the nondominant upper arm. The wounds were measured at regular intervals. This study was the first of its kind and was published in 2005 in the *Journal of Gerontology.* The results made headline news when it was determined that exercise indeed had a significant impact on wound healing. In the exercise group, the average number of days it took the wounds to heal was twenty-nine and in the control group (nonexercisers), the average was forty days.

In this same study, the researchers also measured cortisol levels in the saliva of the participants. Prolonged high cortisol levels, which are associated with stress, tend to slow healing. Physical stress, such as exercise, temporarily raises cortisol levels, and it is believed to be the *regulation* of cortisol by the neuroendocrine system—the ability to release cortisol appropriately rather than have persistently high levels—which enhance immune function. So, in this study, at the three-month evaluation mark, the researchers measured cortisol levels in both groups after they took a treadmill stress test. What they found was that only in the group that had exercised for the past three months was there a significant rise in cortisol. What the scientists who conducted this study concluded was that exercise significantly enhanced wound healing and though they are not sure of how this works, they suggested that there were two logical explanations:

1. Exercise was shown to enhance immune function (the neuroendocrine response measured by cortisol levels). The researchers concluded, "Thus, the data are consistent with the notion that exercise may facilitate wound healing, in part, via neuroendocrine regulation."
2. Exercise also causes blood flow to be accelerated and enhanced. The scientists surmised, "Also, exercise may contribute to blood flow to the skin and increased skin oxygen tension, thereby enhancing wound-healing rates."

Research also suggests that with many conditions, the *overall prognosis improves* with regular physical activity. This means that exercise assists you in healing *and* helps to prevent further medical problems in the future. For example, most people know that there is a very strong link between exercise and preventing a stroke or heart attack. However, many people don't realize that exercise helps to decrease the risk of contracting many other illnesses, including cancer. In medical terms this means that exercise helps to reduce the risk of a primary malignancy (a first or initial cancer). Exercise may also help prevent cancer recurrence in some cases. The most studied cancers for preventing recurrence have been colon, breast, and prostate.

Heart disease, stroke, and cancer are the top three serious medical conditions that people in developed countries are likely to encounter, and exercise is exceedingly important in all of them in terms of physical recovery and the possibility of an improved prognosis. However, exercise also has important prognostic indications in other conditions, including chronic diseases such as fibromyalgia, arthritis, osteoporosis, low back pain, and many others. In the majority of chronic conditions, those affected who exercise regularly and appropriately tend to have a better prognosis and experience less pain and disability.

So, exercise helps you to heal *faster* and *better,* and may *improve your overall prognosis.* Though the research on how exercise facilitates physical healing is still evolving and we don't understand all of the reasons that make this such a potent therapy, we do know that it is a powerful method of encouraging optimal healing. Of course, it makes sense that when you are sick, you become weaker and have less strength and endurance. The rate of muscular decline while on bed rest can be as high as 1 percent to 3 percent per day and after three or more weeks, it's possible for us to lose as much as 50 percent of our strength. But as you can see from the research on exercise and healing, there is much more to this equation than simply regaining strength. Exercise has many profound and wonderful consequences when it comes to recovery.

Make the Most of the Time You Spend Exercising

In the exercise literature there is much discussion about "physical activity" versus "exercise" and whether all physical activity (including such things as mowing the lawn, vacuuming, or walking to the mailbox) should be considered exercise. Rather than enter that debate, what I want to emphasize here are the kinds of physical movements that facilitate optimal physical recovery. If you are running around doing a lot of errands and chores, this is more likely to make you physically fatigued without giving you a lot of healing benefit, whereas, if you spent your time and energy on a more structured exercise plan, you'd likely get greater therapeutic benefit. What this boils down to is, *What are the best ways to exercise to facilitate healing and to avoid excessive fatigue?*

There is no doubt that physical activity is great for people, but a formal therapeutic exercise program will provide you with better results in less time—which means that in order to heal optimally, you would be better off paying someone else to cut your lawn and instead focusing your time and energy on those exercises that will facilitate your recovery. If you are able to have someone else cut your lawn (or perform other physically draining rather than sustaining chores), give yourself permission during the time you are healing to opt out of these activities and focus on the types of exercise that will help you to heal.

Exercise is important in healing, and ideally it involves a planned program that includes setting goals and keeping track of certain parameters such as intensity and time spent doing the activity.

There are many ways to categorize exercises, and in rehabilitation medicine we often break it down into these five categories:

1. Aerobic (also called cardiovascular or endurance) exercises
2. Strengthening exercises
3. Flexibility (also called range of motion or stretching) exercises
4. Functional (also called coordination or balance training) exercises
5. Sport-specific exercises

In physical healing, it is the first two types, aerobic and strengthening, that are usually the most important, though the others may need to be addressed, depending on your specific illness or injury and whether you are an athlete or not. The benefits of these two categories of exercise are listed in Table 10.1.

Flexibility exercises become important in a variety of situations, such as after a woman (or man) has a mastectomy for breast cancer, she may develop shoulder problems that improve with flexibility exercises. People with low back pain may need to work on hamstring flexibility to decrease spinal stress. When it comes to functional exercises, these become important, for example, after someone has a stroke and there are balance and coordination issues. In athletes, working on sport-specific training (such as running sprints or shooting baskets or serving a tennis ball) is essential for optimal recovery. These are just examples of how flexibility, functional, and sport-specific exercises can play a role in healing. However, in general, I recommend that most of the time you allot for exercise be spent on the first two categories, because they are usually by far the most important in physical recovery.

Getting Started

Several reputable organizations, including the American Heart Association and the American College of Sports Medicine, have suggested formal exercise guidelines that include information on when to perform such tests as cardiac stress tests prior to beginning an exercise program. These guidelines are very useful, but they do not address what to do if you are recovering from a serious injury or illness. I encourage everyone to check in with his or her physician about how to safely exercise.

The discussion with your doctor should include what types of exercises you can do, how hard you can push yourself, what you should avoid, and what problems you may encounter and should watch out for. If you have had surgery, your doctor will likely not want you to exercise within a month or so of the operation. Of course, the type of surgery makes a difference. For example, removing a gallbladder with tiny incisions through a laparoscope is very different from having open-heart surgery that involves a big incision and opening the chest and bony sternum. You also will want to talk to your doctor about any symptoms you are having, especially postoperative pain, as that may affect your ability to exercise. Tables 10.5 and 10.6 list when you should stop or avoid exercising.

It's good to have an idea of what your target heart rate should be during aerobic exercise (refer to Table 10.7). A doctor who is guiding a patient in beginning an exercise regimen may opt to do some formal testing such as an electrocardiogram (EKG) or cardiac stress test (usually done on a treadmill or with an upper-extremity bike). The physician may suggest physical or occupational therapy, particularly if someone is very debilitated or has other medical issues such as postoperative musculoskeletal pain, delayed wound healing or scarring, or underlying health problems such as diabetes or heart disease.

If you're going to effectively use physical activity to heal optimally, you'll want to make exercise a habit—something you do regularly without giving it much thought. Starting a new habit takes concentration and planning, but once you have it down, it becomes simple, like brushing your teeth or putting on your seatbelt or reading at night before bed.

Trying to make exercise fun is important. You may enjoy exercising more if you join a class such as yoga or jazz dance. Meeting a friend to go for a walk or run might make it less painstaking to do. It is also important to not feel guilty if you take a day, a week, or even a month off. Guilt leads to stress and stress isn't good for your body or spirit. So, if you stop exercising for a period of time, don't feel guilty or worried about this. Instead, plan a time when you can get back on track and then congratulate yourself for doing so.

Be sure to add some strength training to your regimen. During the 1800s, exercise was thought to be good for the spirit and helped to build character. Some touted it as a moral obligation and the term "muscular Christianity" came into use. While I wouldn't go so far as to say that exercise is a moral obligation, I will say that it will do a lot to help you to heal optimally.

Most people are well aware of the importance of exercise in promoting good health and preventing disease. Physician Robert Levine writes, "The evidence supporting the value of exercise in terms of reducing various diseases and overall mortality is overwhelming to the point that people who avoid physical activity do so at their own peril." However, what people are generally not as aware of is the incredible impact that exercise has on healing.

Healing Strategies

Aerobic Exercise

Walking is a great way to start to exercise and one that has been prescribed since ancient times. Around 400 BC, Hippocrates published a book on preventive medicine called *Regimen in Health* in which he advocated walking, slowly in the summer and quickly during winter months. Over time, walking has been perhaps the most popular form of physical exercise. One reason why walking is a good place to begin is that almost everyone can do this. If you can't walk, refer to Table 10.8 for some other suggestions for aerobic exercise; also, talk to your doctor about what else might be safe for you to try.

In his book *Flow: The Psychology of Optimal Experience*, Mihaly Csikszentmihalyi writes of how walking, a seemingly simple task, offers much in the way of setting goals and achieving them. He comments,

> Walking is the most trivial physical activity imaginable, yet it can be profoundly enjoyable if a person sets goals and takes control of the process . . . A great number of different goals might be set for a walk. For instance, the choice of the itinerary: where one wishes to go, and by what route. Within the overall route, one might select places to stop, or certain landmarks to see. Another goal may be to develop a personal style, a way to move the body easily and efficiently. An economy of motion that

maximizes physical well-being is another obvious goal. For measuring progress, the feedback may include how fast and how easily the intended distance was covered; how many interesting sights one has seen; and how many new ideas or feelings were entertained along the way.

In 2002, snowboarder Chris Klug won a bronze medal at the Winter Olympics. Eighteen months prior to this incredible victory, Klug underwent a life-saving liver transplant, so that he wouldn't suffer the same deadly fate from a condition called primary sclerosing cholangitis that claimed the life of football great Walter Payton. What is remarkable about Klug is not only his amazing athletic prowess, but also his dedication to healing optimally. When I talked to Klug, he told me that the first thing he did after his surgery was to walk around the hospital. After he was discharged, he began a more intense walking program that included touring the city of Denver, where he was temporarily staying to be close to his doctors. Though it may seem trivial, walking is a relatively complex process that helps to improve balance, strength, and endurance throughout the body.

What I recommend is to obtain a pedometer, an inexpensive and simple device to use, and begin to record how many steps you are taking each day. At first, all you are doing is figuring out how active you are during the day. With this as your baseline, you can set a short-term and a long-term goal that involves increasing the number of steps you are taking. Usually, a reasonable initial short-term goal is to increase the average number of steps you are taking by one thousand steps per day. The goal for active healthy people is ten thousand steps per day, so consider this number when you are making your long-term goals. Ten thousand steps per day is not realistic for some people, so I just offer this as a marker of what is a good level for people without any health restrictions. Most people really enjoy wearing a pedometer and many of my patients tell me that is the single best piece of advice that I give them.

Table 10.2 describes some tests that you can perform to establish a baseline for walking. These are fun to do and it's encouraging to retest yourself at a four-week interval and note your progress. You can use one of these tests as your baseline and then set goals based on the results of the test you choose. If you are able to, I encourage you to do at least one of the tests listed in this table.

Strength Training

I know that readers will have various levels of experience with strength training, so I'll offer several suggestions for how to begin (or resume) a strengthening program. Consider these options and choose the one that best fits with your experience level and your current physical condition.

1.   If you have no previous training or you have been through a very serious illness, consider working with a physical therapist.

2.   Another professional you can consult regarding exercise is a personal trainer. Though the credentialing process for trainers is quite inconsistent (which means that the quality of personal trainers can vary widely), finding a knowledgeable trainer can be very helpful. You should look for someone who is interested in your health status and makes adjustments that are appropriate rather than just telling you to "work harder." When my patients get into trouble using a trainer, it is almost always because the trainer doesn't consider the patient's health status and just has a "no pain, no gain" attitude. Look for a trainer who is thoughtful and knowledgeable.

3.   If you have exercised in the past and have a regular strengthening routine, then you can slowly go back to it. Start at a very comfortable level. There is no need to push yourself hard in the beginning. At first, you are just trying to resume your program and let your body get used to doing some strength training. Most people can safely advance by 10 percent (resistance and repetitions) every four weeks or so. You may be able to progress more quickly, but it's always better to take a slow-and-steady path rather than progress too quickly, get injured, and then quit altogether. When it comes to strength training, slow and steady wins the race.

4.   Finally, Table 10.9 lists three very basic strength-training exercises—the first one is for strengthening your arms, the second one is for improving leg strength, and the third one is for core strengthening (your core is the middle of your

body and this supports everything else). These are three very key exercises and extremely easy to do for most people. The idea of doing three strengthening exercises is a great way to get started. These exercises don't cover all the muscle groups, so this won't be a complete program. However, in the beginning the most important thing is to simply get started while avoiding injury. Thus, while this is an abbreviated program, you can begin with these exercises and then tailor your goals around them.

Cross-training

Cross-training is a technique whereby you alternate your exercise routine in order to get the greatest benefit and lessen your risk of injury. For example, swimming is a wonderful form of aerobic exercise, but it doesn't provide the important bone health effects that weight-bearing exercises (such as walking) do. Also, it is not uncommon for swimmers, especially those who don't cross-train, to end up with shoulder problems from overuse. Walking is a great exercise, but doesn't tend to work the upper body as much as it does the lower body. Also, walking is an open chain kinetic exercise so it involves some pounding that other aerobic exercises avoid. Closed chain kinetic exercises, those where your feet are on pedals (such as using a stair stepper or a rowing machine, or cycling), tend to be easier on your joints and back because you avoid the pounding that takes place with open chain exercises (such as walking, running, and skating).

Cross-training not only helps you to get your body in the best shape possible while reducing your risk of injury, it also helps to make your exercise regimen a lot more interesting. So, while I recommend starting with walking and keeping track of your steps, when you feel up to it, add some other types of aerobic exercise to your program. Table 10.8 lists different types of aerobic exercises you can consider.

Table 10.1 Benefits of Exercise

Enhances immune system function

Increases blood volume and improves hemostasis

Enhances strength

Lowers cholesterol levels

Strengthens bones

Increases lean body mass

Improves metabolism

Helps to control blood sugar levels

Improves lean body mass and helps to control weight

Helps to maintain better balance and coordination

Improves heart and lung function

Reduces the risk of serious heart problems

Promotes a positive outlook

Reduces stress, anxiety, and depression

Lessens fatigue

Contributes to better sleep

Reduces the effort to perform work and home activities

Improves sense of well-being

Improves quality of life

Table 10.2 Baseline Walking Tests (Choose One)

Count Your Steps

Buy a pedometer and count your steps for one week. Then take the average daily step count and try to increase this by 10 percent per week. So, if you are currently taking an average of 2,000 steps per day, then your goal for next week would be 2,200 steps per day and a four-week goal might be to advance to 2,800 steps per day. Some people may advance a little slower or faster which is fine. The 10 percent per week rule is just a guideline.

One-Minute or Six-Minute or Twelve-Minute Walk (or Run) Test

To do this, take your pulse for one minute at the beginning and the end of the walk or run. The test is easy and you simply measure how far you can walk (or run) in one, six, or twelve minutes. If you are able to walk for twelve minutes, use that as your time frame. However, if you can't easily walk for twelve minutes, then do this test with either a one-minute or a six-minute time frame. You can do this on a track where you know the distance around the perimeter or you can do the test in your neighborhood, and then drive the same distance using the mileage tracking device to see how far you went. Record your heart rate and how far you were able to go and record this in your log. An initial four-week goal would be to increase

(cont'd)

how far you are able to go in the allotted time by 10 percent over the course of the month. So, if you did the twelve-minute walk test and you were able to go one mile, then your next goal would be to walk 1.1 miles in twelve minutes.

Rockport One-Mile Walk Test

This is a variation on the six- or twelve-minute walk test (you don't need to do more than one walk or run test—the point is to complete a baseline test so you have some data and then you can create goals from that data point and progress appropriately). In this test, you measure your heart rate before and after a mile walk. Time yourself during the walk and then record your heart rate and your time in your log book. As an initial four-week goal, aim to improve your time by 10 percent over the course of the month. So, if you walked the mile in fifteen minutes, then next month's goal would be to walk the mile in one and a half minutes less (or 13.5 minutes).

Table 10.3 Baseline Strength Tests

Push-up Test

This test is done by counting how many push-ups you can do without taking a break. You can either perform the push-ups with your legs straight or with your knees bent and touching the ground. Either way, keep your back straight and avoid touching your belly to the floor as you descend. Your hands should be shoulder-width apart and you should lower yourself until your chin barely touches the ground. Again, a reasonable short-term goal is to increase the number of push-ups you can do by 10 percent over the course of a month. So, if you can do twenty pushups, then your next goal is to do twenty-two.

Sit-up Test

For this test, you will need some masking tape and a metronome. To set the test up, lie on your back on a flat surface with your knees bent at ninety degrees and your arms straight against your sides with the palms face down. Place a piece of masking tape at the tips of your fingers on both sides. Then, measure ten centimeters from these pieces of tape (forward) and place two more pieces of tape there. Set the metronome at fifty beats per minute and while lying on your back, slowly curl forward with the first beat until your fingers reach the second set of taped lines. Then return to lying on your back with the next beat and repeat this for one minute (ideally you do this without pausing, but if you need to pause, that's fine). If you

(cont'd)

complete the test without pausing, you'll have done twenty-five total sit-ups or crunches. You can set a number of different goals with this test, depending on how well you do as a baseline. For example, if you can only do ten sit-ups, then your first short-term goal can be to increase this by five sit-ups over the course of a month. If you can do twenty-five sit-ups, then you can decide to keep going and see how many total sit-ups you can do. Let's say you can do thirty without stopping, then the next month, you might aim to do forty using the metronome to keep time.

Table 10.4 Examples of Exercise Goals

Aerobic

- Obtain a pedometer and keep a log of how many steps you are taking daily. Then, for your first short-term goal, increase this number by five hundred to one thousand steps a day.
- Take a daily walk at a track, in your neighborhood, or at the mall.
- Join a water aerobics class.
- Make a habit of using your stationary bicycle, stair stepper, or elliptical trainer whenever you talk on the phone, and keep track of the minutes.

Strengthening

- Perform the Push-up Test and use this as your baseline. Increase the number of push-ups you can do by 10 percent.
- Perform the Sit-up Test and use this as your baseline. Increase the number of sit-ups you can do by 10 percent.
- Begin your program with the three exercises listed in Table 10.3. Increase the number of each gradually—usually 10 percent every four weeks is reasonable.
- Make an appointment with a physical therapist or a personal trainer to develop an appropriate exercise program for you.

Table 10.5 When to Stop Exercising

Stop Exercising Immediately if you experience*:
- Excessive fatigue or shortness of breath
- Heart palpitations
- Chest, jaw, or arm pain
- Dizziness or light-headedness

*These symptoms should be reported to your doctor.

Table 10.6 When to Skip or Avoid Exercise

Skip or avoid exercise if you:
- Recently had surgery and haven't been cleared by your doctor
- Have any type of infection including a wound infection or upper respiratory infection
- Have uncontrolled pain, nausea, or other treatment side effects
- Feel dizzy or unstable and haven't been cleared by your doctor to exercise with these symptoms
- Have a fever greater than 100 degrees
- Had chemotherapy within the past twenty-four hours (check with your doctor on when to exercise following chemotherapy or other treatments)
- Have low blood cell counts (this is up to your doctor to determine safe levels)

Table 10.7 Target Heart Rate (THR)

It's a good idea to try to keep your heart rate within your target heart rate (THR) range when you exercise. When you start to exercise, you may want to stay close to the beginning of the range, and as you get stronger and have more endurance, you can push yourself a bit harder and work at the end of your range. Record your range in your log, so you can easily refer to it. You can monitor your heart rate by taking your pulse at the wrist or neck. Another inexpensive and fun way to do this is to purchase a heart rate monitor. You can get these at your local sporting-goods store and at many online retailers.

Monitoring Target Heart Rate (THR)
Some general guidelines are that in an untrained individual, an average resting heart rate is usually between 60 and 100 beats per minute. In young adults, the maximal heart rates with exercise are around 190 to 200 and in middle-aged and older adults they are generally 140 to 160. Your THR is what you should aim for when you are aerobically exercising. If you have done some exercise testing, you may have been told your target heart rate or given a range for your target heart rate. If you don't know your target heart rate a simple calculation is as follows:

Maximum Heart Rate (MHR) = 220 − Your Age
Target Heart Rate (Lower Limit) = 0.6 × MHR
Target Heart Rate (Upper Limit) = 0.8 × MHR

Table 10.8 Aerobic Exercises

Aerobics classes on land or in water
Basketball
Cross-country skiing
Cycling
Dancing
Hiking
Jogging
Jumping rope
Rollerblading
Roller-skating or ice-skating
Rowing
Snowshoeing
Soccer
Stair stepper, elliptical, or spinning machines
Swimming
Tennis
Treading water
Walking
Water walking

So, if you are forty years old, then your MHR is 180 (220 − 40 = 180). This means that the lower limit of your target heart rate is 0.6 × 180 = 108 and the upper limit is 0.8 × 180 = 144. You can round these numbers off and use them as your target heart rate range from 110 to 150, which means that you at least try to get your heart rate above 110 but not over 150. Target heart rate goals can be a bit higher in people who are very fit and a bit lower in people who have heart conditions or are on blood pressure medications.

Table 10.9 Three Basic Strengthening Exercises*

Arms
Start with the Push-ups Test and then increase by 10 percent every four weeks.

Legs
Perform a modified squat by sitting in a chair (with or without using your arms for support, depending on if you need to use them) and then rising. Do this ten to fifteen times and then rest for two minutes. Repeat this again and then stop. You can also do this with your back against the wall, pretending to sit in a chair, and then rising.

Core
Perform the Sit-ups Test. Then increase the number by five to ten sit-ups over the course of four weeks.

*You can always progress faster or slower, depending on what feels comfortable to you.

Table 10.10 Exercise Adaptations for Medical Problems

Arthritis

Non-weight-bearing cardiovascular exercises help to avoid stress on the joints. Examples include cycling and swimming. Taking breaks is helpful to minimize pain. Strengthening muscles around painful joints can be done with isometric exercises, which means that there is no movement. Tighten the muscle in the thigh and hold it for six to ten seconds. Open-chain exercises where the foot is not in contact with the floor is one way to exercise the lower extremity without adding stress to the joints, such as when lying on your back and raising one foot about six inches off the ground and holding for thirty seconds.

Diabetes

Cardiovascular exercises may lower blood sugar levels, so it is important to monitor this carefully. Lower load and higher repetition are recommended for strengthening exercises. Be sure there is no chafing or breakdown on your feet caused by sweating.

Back Pain

Lumbar stabilization exercises are recommended to improve core (middle of the body) muscle strength and flexibility. Generally avoid high-load strengthening exercises.

Osteoporosis

Weight-bearing exercises help to strengthen bones. This includes both aerobic and muscle-strengthening exercises. Of note is that swimming and water aerobic exercises, while good for your heart, don't help to strengthen bones because they are non-weight-bearing exercises.

Hypertension

Strengthening is best done with a lower load and higher repetition program while avoiding isometric exercises (which involve a sustained muscular contraction rather than moving through a range). Monitor blood pressure or perceived exhaustion when performing cardiovascular exercises and avoid holding your breath.

Aerobic exercises that avoid or limit leg use:

Swimming
Upper-extremity cycling
Upper-extremity rowing
Water aerobics
Chair aerobics
Cardio punching bag
Upper-extremity circuit training

chapter 11

You Can Sleep to Heal

A doctor who I'll call Joyce came to a conference that I was directing, a couple of hours from our offices. The conference ended in the late afternoon, and we both drove home alone. About twenty minutes into my drive I passed a terrible accident that occurred on the opposite side of the interstate and backed up traffic on that side for miles. The accident was disturbing; it was clear people were seriously injured. Still, I forgot about it when I got home and began making dinner for my kids and getting them ready for bed. The next day, Joyce called and told me that when she was driving home she had somehow crossed over the center barrier on the interstate and had hit a van head-on. The other vehicle had a father and his children in it—everyone was injured. Joyce sustained some bone fractures and skin lacerations; I don't know what happened to the others. Joyce, who was found to be sober at the time of the accident, was criminally prosecuted for reckless driving and part of the prosecution's case centered on the belief that she was overly fatigued. Laws that concern fatigue and car accidents—often called "drowsy driving laws"—vary from state to state but are based on the extensive sleep research that demonstrates how impaired tired drivers are.

Indeed, fatigue can be a criminal offense under the right circumstances—usually when a vehicular or industrial accident occurs that is believed to be caused by someone whose mind and body are not functioning optimally because he or she is tired. Major industrial nuclear catastrophes such as Chernobyl and Three Mile Island, as well as serious accidents including the *Exxon Valdez* and the Space Shuttle Challenger, have been attributed in part to sleepiness in the workplace. When it comes to "drowsy drivers," the article "Fatigue and the Criminal Law," which appeared in *Industrial Health*, notes that most countries and states don't have laws regulating fatigue, but tired drivers who get into accidents can be prosecuted under various other statutes such as "dangerous driving."

The state of New Jersey, recognizing that excessive sleepiness is the second leading cause of car accidents and a major cause of truck accidents in the United States, is more specific and makes it an offense for a person to drive if he or she has not slept in the previous twenty-four hours (the law can be invoked if there is a death caused by the crash or if the accident involves a motor vehicle). Studies have shown that sleepy drivers are just as dangerous as drunk drivers. According to an article titled "Sleep Deprivation," which appeared in the medical journal *Primary Care: Clinics in Office Practice*, "Subjects who drove after being awake for 17 to 19 hours performed worse than those who had a blood alcohol level of .05 percent. Twenty to 25 hours of wakefulness produces performance decrements equivalent to those observed at a blood alcohol concentration of 0.10%, a level deemed unsafe and unacceptable when working or driving."

Sleep is so incredibly important for physical and mental restoration that without proper rest, we don't function well. Optimal physical healing, regardless of the underlying illness or injury, requires excellent sleep. Our bodies know this intuitively. Consider the two things that happen without fail when you have an acute infection: you get a fever and you sleep more. These are the body's natural defenses against infection. But sleeping well does much more than just help fight infection, it helps you to physically heal because a variety of concerted chemical reactions take place when you are least aware of them happening.

Why Good Sleep Helps You Heal

Sleep is a complicated process and there is still much we need to learn about what happens during the time that we rest. All mammals sleep, though in radically different amounts and in various ways. For example, in order to avoid drowning, aquatic mammals sleep on one side of their brain at a time. Humans ideally need to sleep a solid seven to eight hours each night. Our sleep is divided into two main stages: non-rapid eye movement (Non-REM) and rapid eye movement (REM). Non-REM is quiet sleep while REM is more active and that's when you dream. In an ideal situation, approximately 75 percent of that time is spent in Non-REM sleep. Non-REM sleep occurs first and is believed to be the type that has the greatest impact on healing and immune function. Non-REM sleep is further divided into four stages beginning with stage 1, when we just begin to fall asleep and are in between sleep and wakefulness. Then, we advance through the other stages until we reach stage 4 where the brain waves, when measured by special equipment, show the highest level of "slow-wave" activity.

Slow-wave sleep is considered to be the most restorative. One theory behind why slow-wave sleep helps with healing is that your body literally slows down, cools off, and lowers its metabolic demand. This allows your body to literally rest and to replenish energy stores like glycogen. At the end of stage 4 Non-REM sleep, we move into REM sleep and then go through another complete cycle, which lasts about ninety minutes or so. This ninety-minute cycle repeats itself throughout the night. The cycle of sleeping and awakening usually operates over a twenty-four-hour period and this biological clock is what is known as our *circadian rhythm*.

Sleep is thought to serve many functions that are not mutually exclusive. These include conserving energy, restoring tissue, increasing the immune defense, and improving mood. Sleep also facilitates what is called "brain plasticity," which involves encouraging our brains to be agile and facile and to be able to work well, including improving memory and concentration and healing well if injured. Sleep deprivation in healthy people, or what is commonly called "sleep debt" (when you owe your body more sleep than it is getting), alters metabolism during the waking hours and promotes premature aging and can lead to a state that is similar to diabetes. In fact, sleep has such an important effect on glucose metabolism that some studies suggest that certain people may be at higher risk for diabetes if they don't sleep well. In diagnosed diabetics, poor sleep may cause such a significant and persistent issue with glucose control that it may affect the progression of the disease.

During sleep, our bodies function differently than when we are awake. For example, our bodies make a chemical called serotonin, and we know that varying levels of serotonin can affect how we feel. In fact, many of the most popular prescription medications for depression are "selective serotonin reuptake inhibitors," which work by allowing more serotonin to be present in the brain, thus improving mood. The activity of the serotonin in our body changes when we are awake and asleep, and though there is still much to sort out about how sleep affects it and how this in turn affects depression, we know there is a strong link.

The immune system, which is of paramount importance in healing, is compromised by too little sleep, poor sleep quality, or fragmented or interrupted sleep. There are a number of things that we know and much we still have yet to learn. For example, we know that wounds heal more slowly when sleep deprivation occurs. We also know that the brain is the primary organ that is affected by sleep and that the brain releases various chemicals and immune products that directly affect other parts of the body, including the immune system. In a report titled "Neuroimmunologic Aspects of Sleep and Sleep Loss," researchers noted, "The complex and intimate interactions between the sleep and immune systems have been the focus of study for several years. Immune factors, particularly the interleukins, regulate sleep and in turn are altered by sleep and sleep deprivation."

The brain-sleep relationship is extremely complicated and there are many chemical reactions that occur simultaneously during the night hours. For example, during sleep there are changes in the secretion of melatonin. Melatonin, produced in greater quantities at night during sleep, is thought to enhance immune function and healing. You may be wondering if a simple solution is to take a melatonin supplement. It's not quite that easy. At this point, it is impossible to predict how much melatonin you would need to take and whether your body would use it in the same manner as the natural melatonin you produce. Besides, melatonin is just one compound and there are many others that are affected. While buying supplements appeals to a lot of people, the truly "simple solution"—which is highly effective—is to sleep enough and sleep well.

In summary, here are some of the ways that sleep helps us to heal:

- Slows metabolism and conserves energy
- Cools the body and the brain
- Improves immune function
- Replenishes glycogen stores
- Promotes and reorganizes memory

- Rehearses new learning
- Enables emotional adjustment through dreams

What Happens to Sleep
After an Injury or Illness

Many people who need to heal have sleep issues. Research shows that sleep problems often begin or are exacerbated by the hospital environment, which can be a difficult place to rest and recuperate. For example, a report titled "Sleep in the Intensive Care Unit" noted that the average amount of sleep per day a patient gets in the ICU setting is *less than two hours*. Hospitals are noisy places, with the buzz of machines and people, and this accounts for continuous sleep interruptions. In a report by the World Health Organization (WHO), it was recommended that hospital noise levels be no higher than 35dB (decibels) at night to 40dB during the day. However, in one study done on noise levels in a general surgical ward, it was found that during the day they reached 70dB. The lowest noise level recorded was 36dB, which occurred during the midnight to 7:00 A.M. shift. This level was just slightly higher than the WHO's recommended *maximum* nighttime level of 35dB.

Constant interruptions and noisy wards are not the only reasons why people sleep poorly in the hospital. Other reasons may include emotional distress that causes difficulty falling asleep or staying asleep. Pain from injuries or surgical incisions can inhibit proper rest. An inability to ignore and sleep through hot flashes or the urge to urinate can cause frequent awakenings. Medication side effects are commonly associated with complaints of fatigue and poor sleep. Lack of exercise combined with lying and napping in bed most of the day also contribute to a disrupted circadian rhythm and insomnia.

Yet, hospitals are where we often begin to heal and where sleep is absolutely critical. Recently, there have been many new studies released that support promoting a more therapeutic healing environment in the hospitals, and many of these have focused on interventions to improve patients' sleep.

Poor sleep may be due to an underlying medical condition such as sleep apnea, which involves pausing during the respiratory cycle—basically holding your breath while you're asleep. One of my patients is a woman in her forties who was diagnosed with breast cancer several years ago. More than a year prior to her diagnosis, she complained of profound fatigue—a symptom she later attributed to her as yet undetected malignancy. She had surgery followed by chemotherapy and radiation. Not surprisingly, her fatigue worsened, and when I first met with her four years after her cancer diagnosis, her primary symptom was debilitating tiredness that limited every aspect of her life, including work. This patient sought out several doctors' opinions regarding her fatigue and was told that she likely had "cancer-related fatigue." During the course of her workup she had a sleep study, which is an excellent objective measure of what happens during the time that someone is asleep and is a test I highly recommend for people with prolonged symptoms of fatigue. This study showed that she had "mild" sleep apnea. Both my patient and her previous doctors discounted this finding as insignificant. "Why not treat your sleep apnea and see how much better you feel?" I asked her. This patient was truly suffering and immediately liked that idea. She responded well to treatment, which includes a nighttime face mask connected to a type of breathing machine, and while she still felt tired at times, her energy improved remarkably.

Proper rest is essential in all cases of serious illness, but with those undergoing heart surgery, sleep takes on even greater importance and can potentially save lives. Approximately seven out of every ten patients who undergo heart bypass surgery complain of sleep problems in the first few weeks after discharge, and for many of these patients this continues for months. Poor sleep has serious implications in heart patients because it can be associated with increases in high blood pressure and heart rate—both of which cause unnecessary strain on the heart and may put it at risk for further injury.

While there is no doubt that people who experience the sudden onset of serious illness need to sleep well during recovery, proper rest is also important for people who are living with a chronic medical condition. Unfortunately, chronic conditions often lend themselves to wreaking havoc with sleep patterns. For example, in a study evaluating sleep patterns in people with early chronic kidney disease, researchers found that there were sleep disorders present in over 80 percent of those studied. The reasons for this have to do with many physical factors that may include altered blood urea, creatinine, and parathyroid hormone levels, as well as the presence of anemia and problems with blood pressure regulation. In another study appraising the extent of sleep problems in women with systemic lupus erythematosus, more than 50 percent were noted to report moderate to severe sleep impairment. In a study determining the effect of pain on sleep in people with chronic low back pain, the researchers found that there was a 55 percent increase in people reporting sleep problems after pain onset.

Sometimes, sleep problems are associated with other symptoms in a "cluster" pattern. For example, pain, fatigue, and depression may all occur together. A businessman in his thirties was telling me about his recent diagnosis of fibromyalgia. He had a cluster of symptoms including diffuse body pain, fatigue with difficulty concentrating at work, and mild depression. After a very extensive medical workup, his doctor told him to focus on three things: exercise, stress reduction, and sleep. This man traveled constantly and had just been through a divorce where he received part-time custody of his young daughter. He told me that initially he followed his doctor's advice and began to exercise and meditate. However, he still had many symptoms of pain and fatigue, and just generally didn't feel well. Recalling his doctor's advice, he thought about his sleep patterns. He said, "It wasn't unusual that I would stay up until midnight and then get up at 5 A.M. to catch a plane. Even when I wasn't traveling, I didn't pay much attention to getting enough sleep." He began to focus on sleep, and gradually, over a period of months, his symptoms improved. However, it wasn't until he addressed all three of the issues his doctor highlighted— lack of physical activity, too much stress, and poor sleep— that he began to turn the tide of his illness.

In a cluster, because each symptom affects the others, when there is an issue with one, it's more likely that the others will become problematic. They all relate to each other and when one improves, so do the others. Sleeping well is paramount, and it's important not to underestimate its value in healing.

Healing Strategies

One day, I was giving a lecture to a group of physicians. One doctor raised his hand and said, "Nearly all of my patients complain that they are tired. How am I supposed to address this issue as well as take care of their other medical problems in a short office visit?" Though there isn't a simple answer to this question, what I suggested is to ask every patient this one question: *Do you have any problems falling asleep, staying asleep, or sleeping well?* If the answer to this question is yes, then the follow-up questions have to do with what is causing poor sleep and the medical interventions are designed to improve sleep duration and/or quality. Basically what I told this doctor is: *Your patients will never feel good if they don't sleep well.*

One of the first steps to take when treating fatigue is to

recognize any problems with the bodily process that restores our energy—sleep. Some people know they aren't getting enough or the right kind of sleep; others aren't so sure. I routinely ask questions about sleep, naps, daytime fatigue, problems with memory and concentration, and moods during office visits. The answers to questions on these topics can provide important clues about how well someone is resting. One thing I have found is that people are often mistaken about how well they sleep at night. For example, I have had literally hundreds of conversations with patients who have come to their office visit with their sleep partner. When I ask the patient if he or she snores or tosses and turns a lot at night, the answer is often negative. Out of the corner of my eye I would see a surprised look on the partner's face and usually they verbally contradict what was just said. What this means is that by and large, people are not able to accurately report what happens to them at night when they are sleeping.

Even if you can't be absolutely sure of how well you are sleeping at night, one thing you can assess is your daytime level of fatigue. The Epworth Sleepiness Scale is a quick way to determine whether you are unusually fatigued. You can take this test in just a couple of minutes. The questions are listed in Table 11.1. It's important to be extremely honest about how likely you are to fall asleep or the test is not valid. It might be enlightening to ask someone who knows you well how he or she would rate you on the Epworth scale, too, and compare the numbers. The higher the score, the more likely you have some sleep issues that need to be addressed. A normal score is no higher than 6 to 7.

This scale was not designed for people who are going through a serious illness, and you may be thinking that an increased level of fatigue is fairly normal for someone who is trying to heal. That's true, and how fatigued you are can be influenced by a variety of factors including your age, the type of injury or illness, medications or other treatment, your health status before you were diagnosed, how inactive you have become, and how long that inactivity has been present. In order to assess how fatigued someone is while healing, I ask my patients the series of questions that are listed in Table 11.2. Depending on their answers, I may recommend tests to determine whether there is a medical reason for their fatigue.

Another thing I recommend to my patients is to consider giving up their naps (if they take them). While under some circumstances, naps are very helpful in alleviating a sleep debt, they can also interfere with good sleep at night. Sometimes, people get into the habit of napping when they don't really need to. In fact, naps may actually be making it harder for them to get the rest they need. So, unless your medical condition is very debilitating or you have some other reason to nap (such as you are a shift worker), I encourage you to give up sleeping during the day and instead take a couple of rest periods where you don't sleep but you do let your body rest.

It's easy for doctors and patients to be seduced into thinking that fatigue is normal for someone who is trying to heal. This may be true in many cases, but it's important to investigate possible causes of fatigue rather than just assume it's a normal state in a given set of circumstances. As. with any symptom, fatigue deserves thoughtful consideration, and perhaps formal investigation of underlying medical factors that may be contributing to it. What I recommend is to come to the conclusion of fatigue being a normal consequence of someone's particular illness or injury after I have excluded other, potentially treatable, causes. Medical reasons for fatigue are extremely common and it's important not to make erroneous assumptions about the cause of low energy. Tables 11.3 and 11.4 list some of the more common causes of fatigue in someone who is healing and possible medical tests that a doctor might order.

For most people, the goal is fairly simple: *to regularly obtain at least eight hours of quality sleep each night and not to feel unusually fatigued during the day.*

"Sleep hygiene" involves those things that you can do at home to promote good sleep. There are a number of behaviors that interfere with one's ability to sleep (such as drinking caffeinated beverages late in the day) and other habits that help us to relax and experience a better night's rest (such as taking a hot bath or meditating). Things that you can do to promote good sleep are listed in Table 11.6.

Evaluating your sleep hygiene is a good place to start, but it won't solve underlying sleep problems such as sleep apnea or medical issues that contribute to fatigue such as anemia. Therefore, if you find that, despite trying to improve your sleep, you are still having problems, talk to your doctor about this. Though it may seem obvious that talking to your doctor about your sleep and energy level can be helpful, most people don't make the effort to do this. In fact, in a Gallup poll, 70 percent of Americans who claimed to have sleep problems reported that they had never discussed this issue with their doctors. Proper rest is particularly important while you are healing, so it's really worth making the effort to have a specific discussion with your doctor about this topic. Table 11.7 lists some information your doctor will want to know to better assess what might be wrong.

For the best results, I encourage people to approach this subject with their doctors in a way that lets them know this is an issue of real concern. It can be easy for physicians who are managing patients with serious injuries and illnesses to focus their attention elsewhere—such as on how to best treat the underlying disorder. Of course, this makes sense. Office visits are usually rather short and doctors can't spend time addressing every issue. Instead, they typically attend to the most important ones. Healing sleep is important, so in order to get your doctor to really evaluate this, make it easy on him or her. Start with saying something like, "I'm having difficulty sleeping at night and feel very tired during the day. I know that some level of fatigue is normal, but I'd like to talk to you about my symptoms and see if there is something that we can do to help me feel better. In order for you to evaluate this, I brought a list of my symptoms and a list of my current medications including all the over-the-counter drugs and supplements that I am taking."

Your doctor may want to order some tests or she may

want you to adjust your medication regimen. There are a number of ways to approach the problem of poor sleep at night and the best way for you depends on a number of factors that only your doctor can fully evaluate. One question I am often asked is, "If my doctor doesn't find anything wrong, is it better for me to take a sleeping pill than not to sleep well?" The answer when you are trying to heal is "probably." However, this is something that you and your doctor need to decide together.

There are a number of purchasable over-the-counter sleep medications and others that are prescription drugs. Today, there are many more options to help with sleep than in the past. Many of these drugs are quite safe to take compared with, for example, older sleep medications, such as Valium, which can become addictive in susceptible individuals if used long term. Table 11.8 lists many of the commonly used sleep drugs in order to give you a sense of the different options. I am not endorsing any particular one, since that really depends on your specific situation. Your doctor can help you decide whether any of them are appropriate for you to take. While I am not promoting using any one particular sleep medication, I heartily endorse the idea of getting a good night's sleep.

Table 11.1 Epworth Sleepiness Scale

Rate each question by giving it a number from 0 to 3.

- 0—Would never doze
- 1—Slight chance of dozing
- 2—Moderate chance of dozing
- 3—High chance of dozing

Questions:

- How likely are you to doze if you are sitting and reading?
- How likely are you to doze if you are watching television?
- How likely are you to doze if you are sitting inactive in a public place (for example, church)?
- How likely are you to doze if you are a passenger in a car for an hour without a break?
- How likely are you to doze if you are lying down to rest in the afternoon (when circumstances permit)?
- How likely are you to doze if you are sitting and talking to someone?
- How likely are you to doze if you are sitting quietly after lunch (without alcohol)?
- How likely are you to doze if you are in a car stopped in traffic for a few minutes?

Table 11.2 Questions I Ask My Patients about Fatigue

- Do you have any problems falling asleep, staying asleep, or sleeping well? Do you feel tired when you awaken in the morning?
- Do you have a sense of feeling unusually tired despite rest?
- Is sleep or rest restorative for you?
- Are you a restless sleeper?
- Do you have difficulty falling asleep or falling back to sleep?
- Do you snore?
- Do you rest or nap during the day?
- Have you curtailed or modified your activities due to your energy level?
- Is fatigue affecting your home life, work, or recreation?
- Do you have difficulty with memory, concentration, attention, or word finding?
- Is your energy level considerably different from what it was before you became ill? If so, in what ways?

Table 11.3 Common Causes of Sleep Problems during Healing

- Alcohol (either excessive use or prescription drug–alcohol interactions)
- Anemia
- Anxiety
- Deconditioning
- Depression
- Glucose (sugar) or hormonal imbalances
- Infection
- Medication or other treatment side effects
- Pain
- Side effects from over-the-counter drugs or "natural" remedies
- Sleep disorders (such as sleep apnea)
- Stress (physical or emotional)

Table 11.4 Screening Tests that May Be Done in a Fatigue Workup

Laboratory Blood Tests
- Complete blood count
- Erythrocyte sedimentation rate
- Creatinine and urea nitrogen
- Glucose
- Calcium and phosphorus
- Electrolytes
- Albumin and total protein
- Liver function tests
- Thyroid function tests
- Rheumatology screen
- C-reactive protein
- Viral titers (such as Lyme, HIV, Epstein-Barr, and the like)

Other Laboratory Tests
- Urinalysis
- Chest X-ray
- Echocardiogram and/or electrocardiogram
- Sleep study

Table 11.5 Example of Goals

Short-term

- Avoid all caffeinated beverages after 1 P.M.
- Reduce wine consumption from one to two glasses in the evening to one or less than one glass.
- Make an appointment to talk to your doctor about fatigue and sleep.
- Review your medications with your pharmacist and determine which ones may affect sleep (either have sedative side effects or the opposite).
- Give up taking naps during the day.
- Plan a fifteen- to thirty-minute rest period daily.

Long-term

Your long-term sleep goal is to regularly sleep, and with good sleep quality, seven to eight hours each night. This should be a six-month goal, and if you aren't able to achieve that in six months, then continue with your short-term goals and repeat the long-term goal for the next six months. I recommend that if you aren't able to meet this goal in the first six months, you check with your doctor about the possibility of having a sleep study.

Table 11.6 The Rules of Good Sleep Hygiene

Manage Your Bedtime Routine
- Go to bed only when you are tired.
- Use your bedroom for sleep and intimacy only (for example, not to watch television).
- Have a relaxing bedroom environment that is at a moderate temperature, quiet, and dark.
- Try to establish a regular bedtime and time you awaken in the morning.
- Develop a bedtime routine that you follow.
- Plan to get seven to eight hours of sleep at night.
- Get rid of your bedroom clock (or hide it if you need the alarm for the morning).
- Get out of bed and go to another room if you are unable to sleep after twenty to thirty minutes (estimate this).

Avoid Things that Interfere with Sleep
- Don't eat a heavy meal before bed, especially one high in sugar.
- Avoid drinking a lot of fluids.
- Stop drinking caffeine at least four to six hours before bedtime.
- Eliminate nicotine before bedtime.
- Avoid alcohol after dinner (four to six hours before bedtime).
- Try not to exercise within two hours of bedtime (some say six hours).

(cont'd)

- Don't watch television or play computer games before bed.
- Avoid naps during the day.
- Be aware that sleeping pills are often only effective when used for a short period of time (two to four weeks) and that some sleeping pills can actually make sleep worse.

Try These Things to Help You Relax Before Bed

- Take a hot bath (not a shower), which may promote sleep.
- Have a light bedtime snack, such as a glass of warm milk or a bowl of cereal.
- Allow at least an hour before bedtime to unwind—take a hot bath, read a book, or listen to music.
- Practice relaxation techniques, such as biofeedback, meditation, deep breathing, or imagery.

Table 11.7 Information to Give Your Doctor

- A list of all of your medications, including over-the-counter drugs you take
- A list of all of the supplements you take
- A list of your symptoms (for example, include when you are tired, whether you snore, how fatigue is impacting your ability to function)
- A description of your mood
- Your alcohol and caffeine consumption
- Your sleep schedule (what time you go to bed, how long it takes you to fall asleep, whether you awaken during the night, and why and what time you get up in the morning)
- A description of your activity level during the day
- Information about naps

Table 11.8 Medications for Sleep*

Over-the-Counter
- Nytol QuickCaps
- Simply Sleep
- Sleepinal Maximum Strength Softgels
- Sominex Maximum Strength Caplets
- Tylenol PM
- Unisom SleepGels
- Unisom SleepTabs

Prescription
- Ambien
- Ambien CR
- Benzodiazepines, such as estazolam (ProSom) or flurazepam (Dalmane)
- Lunesta
- Rozerem
- Sonata

*Other medications may be used to help with sleep as well. For example, muscle relaxants or antidepressants can have sedating effects while also treating underlying muscle spasms or mood disorders, respectively.

Alcohol's Effect on Sleep

Some people will use alcohol as a method of relaxation and even a sleep aid. Alcohol does not do either of these things well. While it may initially relax you, it tends to act as a depressant and affects your mood negatively. Dr. Lawrence Epstein, a sleep expert, dispels the myth that alcohol is helpful in getting people to sleep in his book *The Harvard Medical School Guide to a Good Night's Sleep*. He calls alcohol the "wolf in sheep's clothing" and cautions "alcohol is not an effective sleep aid. Its sedative effect may make you fall asleep faster, but it has a harmful effect on sleep quality that far outweighs this benefit."

chapter 12

You Can Use Spirituality or the Universe to Heal

A woman I met at a talk I gave to a group of cancer survivors told me she had been diagnosed with cancer in the 1970s. At that time, she was told she had less than six months to live and she opted for very aggressive treatment that lasted over four years and included twenty-eight surgeries or other procedures (including bone marrow transplantation). Her husband tried valiantly to keep her spirits up during treatment and he hung a sign over the door to their home that read something like "If you are going to cry, please leave! We need encouragement and hope." He then went around the house and posted Bible verses in every cabinet, so when she opened them, that's the first thing she saw. Fortunately, she survived, but her illness was a harrowing experience and, not surprisingly, it took its toll on her physically, emotionally, and spiritually.

We are complex beings, and our lives are filled with many relationships and influences. The "healing landscape" of our lives can be viewed as those people and things that are meaningful to us and exert a positive influence. For some, the healing landscape may include a "religious sanctuary," and God or a Creator. For others, healing energy may come from nature or the Universe.

Spiritual scholars have come up with various definitions about the difference between religion and spirituality. Spirituality is often defined as believing in that which is "sacred or holy." This is usually coupled with a transcendent (greater than self) relationship with God or another higher power or a universal energy. The National Institute of Health Care Research convened a panel of experts who defined spirituality as "the feelings, thoughts, experiences, and behaviors that arise from a search for the sacred." Religion, on the other hand, is more formal and involves a specific set of beliefs, rituals, and practices that are often culturally ingrained. Spirituality is amorphous whereas religion has more borders and definition

People who are spiritual do not necessarily believe in God or another deity. Instead, spirituality can be expressed in other ways such as through a connectedness with nature. While believing in God is not a prerequisite for a spiritual life, the vast majority of people in the United States (at least 95 percent) do believe in God or a higher spiritual power. In *Who Needs God,* Rabbi Harold Kushner writes:

> [T]here are no atheists in foxholes and few atheists in hospitals. It is not because people are hypocrites, ignoring God when things are going smoothly and suddenly discovering Him and pleading piety when they are in trouble. And it is not just a matter of turning to God out

of fear. There are no atheists in foxholes because times like those bring us face to face with our limitations . . . People have always found God at the limits of their own strength.

Many people also believe that God acts through physicians and other healthcare providers to help people heal. In one study conducted in the southeastern region of the United States, 80 percent of respondents said they believed God acts through physicians to cure illness. In another study conducted in Pakistan, 92 percent of the people studied said they thought that doctors had healing powers given by God.

Congregational rabbi Samuel Karff notes that in biblical and rabbinic Judaism there have always been three partners in the healing of the sick. God is the ultimate healer. There is often a "human agent or partner" who helps facilitate healing. Then, the third partner is the ill person himself. Rabbi Karff explains that in this tradition, "proper self-care begins with a recognition that one cannot be physician to one's self, but the patient remains as an active partner with God and the human healer in responding to illness."

Faith is defined as a belief in something for which there is no proof. *Prayer,* though usually thought of in a religious context, can be associated with nonreligious aspects of spirituality such as meditation. Of note is that these definitions are the subject of great debate, and many religious scholars make a clear distinction between meditation and prayer. Both prayer and meditation may be helpful healing resources, and you can consider using one or the other or both if they appeal to you. Whatever helps you and makes you feel better—peaceful and hopeful—is the right thing to do.

As a cancer survivor, I am often asked by those who are newly diagnosed what really helped me get through the experience. Hearing this question over and over and knowing how much it helped me to talk to cancer survivors who were several years ahead of me in their survival, I decided to write a book on this topic. *What Helped Get Me Through: Cancer Survivors Share Wisdom and Hope,* was published by the American Cancer Society after I interviewed more than two hundred cancer survivors and compiled their responses. One of the questions I included on the survey was, "Did religion or spirituality help you cope with cancer?" Not surprisingly, I received many different responses.

Some of the people who responded thought that formal religion played a part in their healing:

> I prayed the Rosary nightly. I learned to be more patient and to let go of things over which I have no control. Before cancer I had to be in charge—I was making the plans—I was taking control. Now I take care of my family and myself and let go of those little things that don't really matter—the dust on the furniture will still be there tomorrow. I put more things in God's hands. I tell people that family, good medicine, and faith got me through the surgery and nine months of treatment.
>
> —*Dorinda, retired teacher, diagnosed with*
> *ovarian cancer at age forty-nine in 2005*
> *in Edison, New Jersey*

I was never a religious person, but I must say, I actually
felt very good when I went to synagogue. I felt connected,
like I was doing yet another thing to help myself.

—Laura, unemployed psychiatric social worker,
diagnosed with breast cancer at age forty-three
in 2006 in Avon, Connecticut

Others mentioned prayer as a way of tapping into their
spirituality:

Prayer, prayer, and more prayer. You have to believe in
something or someone to help you get through the cancer
ordeal.

—Debra, administrative assistant, diagnosed
with ovarian cancer at age fifty-one
in 2007 in Chicago, Illinois

I am not a particularly religious person, but my family is,
and I did find it comforting when people told me that they
were praying for me or that I was in their prayers. It was
also comforting to receive little medals or prayer cards.

—Todd, oncology social worker, diagnosed with
chronic myelogenous leukemia at age twenty-five
in 1997 and kidney cancer at age thirty-three
in 2005 in Warwick, Rhode Island

Some cancer survivors said that spirituality helped
them to have a positive attitude or to feel more relaxed or
focused:

Spirituality did help me. It made my mind stronger by allowing me to concentrate on my fight.

> —*Jitendra, software engineer, diagnosed with*
> *non-Hodgkin's disease at age twenty-seven*
> *in 1994 in Cleveland, Ohio*

I am not a religious person, but I am a spiritual one. When I found out I was ill, I renewed my interest in the Buddhist philosophy, finding it very calming and reassuring. I do not fear death or what may come afterward.

> —*Judy, retired accounting clerk, diagnosed with*
> *lung cancer at age sixty-four in 2004*
> *in Norwalk, California*

Although I am Jewish by birth, I do not observe any religious rituals or beliefs. I did regularly see a "hands-on healer"—a wonderful woman who would bring me such peace through the calm placement of her hands. Although I didn't totally believe that she was healing my body through her hands, I *did* believe that laying on of her hands brought my body and soul true peace and calmness.

> —*Elena, arts administrator, diagnosed with*
> *inflammatory breast cancer at age forty-four*
> *in 1999 in Silver Spring, Maryland*

Faith. My motto during my entire cancer experience was and still is 'Faith and Humor.' I even had this tattooed with the colon cancer ribbon on my ankle. I went to Las Vegas and had it (the tattoo) done two days after my chemo doc said I was cancer-free. I knew I was a survivor from the day my cancer was diagnosed. The Lord made it very clear to me that this road was not going to be easy, but that I would make it to the end.

—*Susan, housewife, diagnosed with colorectal cancer*
at age forty-three in 2006 in
Mobile, Alabama

Some individuals found strength in nature or the Universe:

I appreciated quiet times with nature, contemplating life and life cycles.

—*Kirsten, distribution assistant, diagnosed with*
colon cancer at age forty-nine in 2006 and endometrial (uterine)
cancer at age fifty in 2007 in Buford, Georgia

I have become open to spiritual insights and beliefs. I now ask for help from the Universe instead of trying to manage everything myself. Before breast cancer, I thought that was all very hippie-ish and just not me at all!

—*Pearl, nurse, diagnosed with breast cancer at*
age thirty-three in 2004 in Glasgow, Scotland

I am not a religious person (I guess that's the scientist in me), but I do believe in a greater good that brings people together. Call it a Zen state or whatever, but finding some sort of inner peace can go a long way.

—*Federico, cancer chemical biologist, diagnosed with*
testicular cancer at age thirty-one in 2006 in
Brookline, Massachusetts

There were also those who really didn't find it helpful to tap into any spiritual or Universal energy:

My mother is religious and brought [to me] one church-man after the other and one pressure group after the other. No thanks.

—Suza, investor relations, diagnosed with
mantle cell lymphoma at age thirty-nine in 2005
in Johannesburg, Gauteng, South Africa

Religion had no part for me. A lot of well-meaning people said they were praying for me, I always thanked them and [did so] from my heart, but it is not for me.

—Matt, carpenter, diagnosed with chronic lymphocytic
leukemia at age fifty in 2003
in Bath, New York

My rabbi would visit; however, truthfully, I didn't find his visits comforting. I still question how a god can let people suffer from things like cancer or Alzheimer's.

—Eileen, technology specialist, diagnosed with
breast cancer at age thirty-four in 1984, acute myelogenous
leukemia at age forty-nine in 1999, and basal cell carcinoma
(skin cancer) at age fifty-five in 2005
in Framingham, Massachusetts

These comments highlight how we all have our own unique perspective on spirituality and healing. Whether you tap into a higher power to help you heal is your decision.

Medical Miracles

Sometimes, people equate religion or spirituality with healing miracles. As a physician, I have seen some truly amazing things happen to people, but what one sees portrayed in the media and what occurs in real-life hospital beds is often very different. The stories that reporters love to document are those featuring people who face tremendous adversity but then go on to heal with seemingly no lasting effects. The media touts these people as heroes who inspire us with their monumental achievements. One of the most well-known media heroes is Lance Armstrong, who was diagnosed with testicular cancer that had spread to his brain. Lance went through cancer treatment and recovered incredibly well— becoming a legend as a cyclist in the Tour de France. He has also done incredible work in the cancer community, and I think the media's positive portrayal of him is hard won and well deserved.

But what happens when the end result isn't a series of Tour de France victories? What happens to guys like Joe Theismann, who don't heal completely? As you may recall, Washington Redskins' quarterback Joe Theismann was voted the National Football League's Most Valuable Player in 1983. His phenomenal twelve-year professional football career came to an abrupt halt on a Monday night in 1985 when New York Giants' defensive lineman, Lawrence Taylor, tackled him. In an interview published in a book titled *Rising to the Challenge*, Theismann describes what happened:

I handed the ball to John Riggins, he turned around and pitched it back to me as he ran toward the line of scrimmage. When I caught it, I looked downfield. I was supposed to throw a deep post-pattern to one of my wide receivers but the safety wasn't fooled. So I was looking for the secondary receiver and I couldn't quite locate the tight end who was supposed to be on the right side. And then I felt some pressure coming from my left side. So I thought I'd step up into the pocket for safety. And as it turns out, Lawrence Taylor grabbed my left shoulder. I was standing rigid in the pocket with my feet firmly planted, and as he swung around, his thigh caught my right leg between my ankle and my knee, and just snapped my leg like a toothpick. And I remember hearing a "pow, pow." It sounded like two muzzled gunshots. It was actually my leg breaking!

Though injuries often end athletic careers, Theismann and his teammates and coaches all hoped that he would fully recover, and initially, it looked like he would. Theismann talks about how he worked at healing:

When I first started therapy, and got out of the cast, I was pleased by the amount of progress I was making. I did everything the doctors and trainers prescribed for me. I would take it to the max, as far as the therapy would go. I would not only work on my leg but work on the rest of my body so that when my leg was healed every part of me would be in good shape. The early part of recovery was really encouraging because I could see large amounts of improvement.

Then after about six or seven months, the improvements started decreasing. The increments were much smaller, still fairly noticeable, but much smaller . . . I started to try and do football-type movements . . . Then all of a sudden, I realized I had lost about 20 percent strength in my right leg. No matter how hard I worked, no matter what I did, I was still unable to get back to the strength that I had.

Theismann was still a tremendous athlete even after his injury, but he wasn't able to resume playing professional football. He said, "Emotionally, for me, I think the toughest times came after leaving the game. While I was still training, while I was still fighting through it, I'd get so frustrated. I'd get so frustrated at times when I was training. I'd cry. And throw things. I was not a very pleasant person to be around because, hell, I wanted to be well. I wanted to play."

I have no doubt that Theismann healed optimally, but as he learned, it is not always possible to heal perfectly. Knowing what to accept and what not to is often very difficult to define. Talk to your doctors about your expectations and theirs. Keep in mind that many patients exceed their doctors' expectations through hard work and determination.

Interestingly, Theismann, who has gone on to do many wonderful things with his life including motivational speaking, has this philosophy: "Most people look at what happened to me as a tragedy in sports. I look at it as a blessing for a man."

Healing Strategies

The word *health* is derived from the Anglican word *Hal*, which means "to be whole or holy." Though there are many ways to use spirituality as a healing resource, all spiritual encounters involve quieting one's mind and working to feel more connected to nature, God or some other deity, or simply an energy source.

For most of history, nearly all healing was entrenched in the spiritual. With the recent establishment of scientific medicine (evidence based treatments), there became a clear delineation between faith and science. As this line was drawn, there were experts on both sides who argued vehemently for their views. Today, there seems to be room to compromise. Patients can experience the tremendous benefits of science and spirituality and "integrate" them into the same healing experience. Religious scholar Martin Marty writes of this changing view:

> Theorists, scientists, practitioners, and patients, on one side, have come to be more open to the voices of faith and the spiritual searches for well-being. Meanwhile, on the other side, theologians, religious philosophers, pastors, and ordinary believers, discerning such openness, have grown friendlier to science."

Not everyone is open to the idea that spirituality can or should help people with physical healing. In the book *Heal*

Thyself: Spirituality, Medicine, and the Distortion of Christianity, two scholars take this stance. The book flap sums up their views in this manner: "*Heal Thyself* argues that our popular culture's fascination with the health benefits of religion reflects not the renaissance of the world's great religious traditions but the powerful combination of pervasive consumer capitalism and a deeply self-interested individualism. A faith-for-health exchange, say the authors, serves to misrepresent and devalue the true meaning of faith."

The study of how healing and spirituality intersect is in its infancy, though the early data is interesting. For example, one study that measured a positive immune response (increased IgA levels) in students found that those who viewed a religious film had significantly higher levels than those who watched a war film. In another study, that measured biologic markers of inflammation such as interleukin-6 (in this case, lower levels being more advantageous) found that of the more than 1,700 people studied, those who attended religious services regularly were more than 40 percent less likely than nonattendees to have high levels of interleukin-6. Other studies have had similar results suggesting that immune system function and healing can be influenced by spirituality.

Studies that have focused on the effect of spirituality and religion on physical health have shown a positive relationship that results in lower blood pressure and blood levels of fat (lipids), enhanced immune function and even longer life span. However, there is much that isn't known about spirituality and healing. In a review article titled "Spiritual Role In Healing. An Alternative Way of Thinking," the authors summarized the current research in this field of medicine by noting, "The link between religion and health is established firmly. What remains tentative is whether it is causal, and, if so, by which mechanisms does it work? Many possible mechanisms may play a role, such as lower rates of drug and alcohol abuse, improved stress management, and enhanced social support."

One of the researchers whose work led to the establishment of the study of psychoneuroimmunology is Candace Pert. Dr. Pert is a former research professor at Georgetown University School of Medicine and section chief at the National Institute of Mental Health who explains her stance on science and spirituality in this manner:

> I'm a scientist viewing the realm of the spirit, approaching it with hardcore, observable evidence; and from the data I've seen, I can no longer deny the existence of God . . . In the matter of science and God coming together, I'm in good company with another scientist, one much more famous and influential than myself: Albert Einstein. His professional journey brought him to a personal epiphany in which he proclaimed that the more he understood the universe, the more he believed that a Creator was at work.

However, though there are many cases one can cite that involve abuses of spirituality, prayer, and religion, when used and practiced with a keen regard for morality, kindness, and peace-seeking they can be helpful resources in healing. In fact, in a study published in *The Journal of Family Practice* titled "Allowing Spirituality into the Healing Process," the author summarized the research on the positive/negative effects of religiosity and its health benefits in this manner:

> In general, research shows the impact of religion and spirituality is positive. Although a person's spirituality is sometimes pathological, and spiritual beliefs can create health issues, an overwhelming number of studies show a positive benefit . . . [In studies] where the impact of spirituality could be classified as positive, negative, no association, complex or mixed, 70 percent showed a positive impact . . . while only 5 percent showed a negative impact. The studies show spirituality and religion benefit patients by helping prevent illness, increasing the ability to cope, and improving outcomes.

Religion, in its most advantageous form to assist with healing, enhances spirituality often through formal rituals and practices. For example, from a Christian perspective Francis Mac-Nutt has written several books on prayer and healing. In *The Power to Heal*, he discusses the sacrament of the sick and notes that when this ritual is administered it helps to "build up the faith" of the ill person and assist her in spending time praying.

When it comes to praying (or meditating, which some individuals may prefer to use instead of prayer or together with it), some people aren't sure how to get started. However, the nice thing about these practices is that when it comes to healing, there is no "right way" to do them. Any way that you decide to pray or meditate will be just fine.

Another way to feel connected is to take a walk outside where you can enjoy nature. This is soothing and helps your body to relax. Almost everyone who takes the time to sit in a beautiful place, near the ocean, in the woods, on a park bench, or anywhere that is peaceful and serene, will be able to utilize this experience in a way to help them heal. The world is a magnificent place to experience; use it to help you recover.

If you are more adventurous and you're able to, do things that have a peaceful and reflective component. One journalist who interviewed me told me that when she was recovering from cancer treatment herself, she decided to train to climb a mountain in Colorado. She described both the training and the actual climb in a very spiritual context—one that involved connecting with nature and a higher power. I have also talked to many people who have planned spiritual vacations to India, Israel, Rome, and other wonderful places.

Making plans to climb a mountain or travel to the Vatican or Jerusalem can be incredibly fulfilling, but so can simply enjoying the opportunities that present themselves on a daily basis. For example, one day I was meeting friends for dinner in the North End (the Italian section) in Boston. As we were walking to the restaurant, we passed a beautiful historic Catholic church. On the spur of the moment we decided to go inside. The church's architecture and stained glass windows combined with hundreds of candles flickering in the semi-darkness were just breathtaking. Visiting any religious sanctuary gives me a sense of peace. I love the quiet, people only talking in hushed tones. I like to take in the beauty and the symbols—whatever they are. Whether it is a simple place or an ornate one, I find these peaceful places to visit.

I also love to go to wide open places where nature abounds and the man-made changes to the environment are limited. Going to parks where there are children happily playing and where I can walk and exercise or sit and watch the kids is also an activity that brings me peace, joy, and hope. These are all emotions that help fuel healing. They can be elusive when you are trying to heal. Think about what works for you—where are your favorite places to be? What helps you to quiet your mind and reflect? What gives you energy and a sense of peace? Tapping into the Universe, nature, spirituality, or your religion may offer you a respite from turmoil.

Your Healing Journey

chapter 13

You Can Overcome Setbacks

"*Next week there can't be any crisis.* My schedule is already full." Henry Kissinger said this in jest, but wouldn't it be great if we really could clear our schedules of disruptions and just focus on healing? Moreover, it would be even better if healing occurred exponentially or even linearly in a straight upward slope, all forward progress with no setbacks or plateaus to discourage us. However, just as Kissinger couldn't avoid dealing with constant governmental crises, neither can we heal without facing impediments, stumbling blocks, or even reversals. This is because *normal healing involves setbacks and plateaus.*

This is a surprise to many people, but not to doctors. Physicians are constantly helping patients overcome healing setbacks and plateaus, and because they are so familiar with them, they may not always recognize how discouraged patients feel when this happens. Essentially, what doctors take for granted and assume is "par for the course" for a particular illness or injury, might be incredibly disheartening to the person experiencing it.

We expect setbacks in most other areas of life. For example, baseball commissioner Francis "Fay" Vincent said in a speech he gave to university students, "Baseball teaches us, or has taught most of us, how to deal with failure. We learn at a very young age that failure is the norm in baseball and, precisely because we have failed, we hold in high regard those who fail less often—those who hit safely in one out of three chances and become star players." Striking out in baseball and in other areas of life doesn't mean that the end result will be failure. The classic example is Babe Ruth, a home run record setter, who also held the record for the most strikeouts. Consider these other legendary setbacks:

- Henry Ford neglected to put a reverse gear in his first car. He failed and went broke five times before finally succeeding.
- The Duke of Wellington's mother considered him a dunce and at Eton, where he was educated, he was called dull, idle, and slow. At age forty-six he defeated Napoleon.
- Legendary poet Robert Frost was told in a curt note by an editor of *The Atlantic Monthly*, "Our magazine has no room for your vigorous verse."
- *Harry Potter and the Philosopher's Stone* was rejected many times before J. K. Rowling finally found a small London publisher willing to accept the book. *Gone With the Wind* was rejected thirty-eight times before becoming a bestselling book and movie. John Grisham had a similar experience with his first novel, *A Time*

to Kill. Dr. Seuss was told that his style was "too different" from other children's books and wouldn't sell.

Life is filled with setbacks and plateaus, but as these examples reveal, the final outcome is not necessarily determined by impediments in the process. Of course, the goal in healing is to try and avoid or limit physical setbacks, but this isn't always possible. Thus, it's helpful to anticipate them and to acknowledge that this is simply part of mending.

There is no doubt that it is terribly discouraging to be working on healing and then to have a setback. However, recognizing the fact that physical and emotional setbacks are normal during recovery helps one to avoid becoming too discouraged.

Why Setbacks Occur

There are two types of setbacks—physical and psychological. Both types may occur for a variety of reasons. Sometimes you can deal with them on your own at home and other times you will need to talk to your doctor about what to do next. It's common and quite normal for people to also experience healing plateaus, where they neither progress nor retrogress. Healing plateaus can occur due to the same reasons that setbacks may occur and can be overcome in a similar fashion.

Physical setbacks may occur when people try to rush

the healing process, and they are too active too soon. For instance, one of my patients was recovering from back surgery. He went on a walk with his girlfriend, but about halfway through he began to feel pain in his back. Instead of staying where he was and having her run home to get the car, he ignored the pain and finished the walk. A few hours later, he was in excruciating agony and his girlfriend called me in tears, asking what could be done. I asked her to put him on the phone and reassured my patient that this would probably just be a minor setback—easily overcome in a few days with rest and medication. However, I also told him that pushing himself physically without regard for his pain level was not a good idea in this early healing phase. I urged him to pay close attention to what his body was telling him and to let that voice help dictate what he was safely able to do.

On the other hand, it's impossible for anyone to predict exactly when it's okay to return to specific activities. Even experienced doctors can only estimate the healing process and when it is safe to resume one's usual activities. While it's good to be careful, being overly cautious and afraid to do what you enjoy doing can also lead to problems associated with inactivity including physical deconditioning and emotional frustration or even depression. As Sophia Loren once said, "Mistakes are part of the dues one pays for a full life."

Psychological setbacks are often difficult to predict but may be relatively easy to address. For example, I wrote an article in *Newsweek* about one type of psychological setback that I frequently see occur in people who are trying to heal. I call these "emotional ambushes." The way an emotional ambush works is that you are going along in your usual state of mind and you hear something or read something that is very disturbing. Your mood plummets, because you worry about this new information, even though it doesn't really affect you directly. For example, when the late Elizabeth Edwards announced to the world that her cancer had spread, many women with a history of breast cancer began to worry about their own cancer spreading. Edwards's news shouldn't really have impacted them, but they were "emotionally ambushed."

When I wrote about emotional ambushes and how they affect healing in *Newsweek*, many readers wrote to me and told me how I had put words to something that they have experienced. It happens to all of us—even people who don't need to heal. For some reason, we begin to "own" news that isn't really something we can do anything about. Of course, we want to feel empathy, but it isn't helpful to us to take that news personally.

One of the best ways to deal with an emotional ambush is to simply recognize it for what it is. Once you recognize an emotional ambush, you can gently put your thoughts and feelings into perspective.

Perspective is important as you encounter healing plateaus and setbacks. It is helpful if you can look at them as offering feedback, rather than suggesting failure.

Healing Strategies

There are several things that will help you to cope with and even overcome healing setbacks and plateaus. The first and perhaps most important step is to simply recognize that they are a normal part of the healing process and that most likely you can still recover well despite them.

While I can offer you some general reassurance on this issue, the more educated you are about your condition, the better you will be able to avoid setbacks and to mentally prepare for them if they do occur. Your best resource is your health-care team. Ask your doctor any questions that you have. He or she will hopefully provide answers that help to alleviate uncertainty. Other health-care professionals can also be extremely helpful and are terrific resources.

In many instances you can avoid psychological setbacks or at least limit the damage that they can cause. One of the best ways to do this is to try and anticipate what might happen and then be prepared for this. I don't mean that you should worry about having every possible side effect from a medication or a procedure. Rather, what I'm saying is to have a realistic expectation of how long it will take you to heal and what you can expect during that time.

For example, when I give talks to people recovering from cancer treatment, invariably I find that many people don't have realistic expectations for how long it will take them to heal after undergoing chemotherapy or radiation or other therapies. For the majority of cancer patients, the recovery period is measured in months to years rather than weeks. But, I often have people come up and tell me, "It's been six weeks, and I still feel terrible." Reassuring them that they will feel better but that it will take much longer than six weeks helps them to put things in the proper perspective and not become overly discouraged.

As mentioned earlier, the key to dealing with emotional ambushes is to simply recognize them. Well-meaning friends can inadvertently ambush someone who is trying to heal. I can't even recall how many people have told me worst-case cancer stories. Though I try to be polite, for my own sanity's sake, I usually try to gently cut people off before they get too far into them.

Whenever I feel ambushed, I remind myself that people are generally kindhearted and may be telling me something that is painful for me to hear because they are suffering themselves. Nevertheless, it's good to recognize what they said as an ambush and put it into the proper perspective. For instance, if someone tells me a worst case cancer story, I tell myself that they are not talking about me, and that my situation is in no way connected to whatever they are sharing.

The media is also a source of potential ambushes. While sometimes news reports offer information about promising new treatments, they too often focus on tragic stories that can ambush people. Remember that news stories go by the motto "if it bleeds it leads." This can lead to many unnecessary ambushes while you are focused on healing. Recognize ambushes for what they are and know that they usually don't apply to your situation. If you find your mood plummeting, ask yourself whether the information you just heard is truly applicable to you or is it simply an inadvertent ambush?

Assess your own expectations. Are they realistic? What is the best way to achieve them? Unrealistic goals can make you feel like a failure when in fact you may be healing quite well. It's not always easy to determine realistic goals, however. The brilliant writer Alice Walker offers us some excellent advice when she tells us to "plan but don't plan as if it will all happen as you planned it." Therefore, if you have experienced a setback or a healing plateau, review your goals and decide whether they need to be revised a bit.

Sport psychologist Jim Taylor also shared with me a terrific piece of advice that he uses with competitive athletes who sustain serious injuries. Dr. Taylor says that he counsels athletes to think about "the here and now and then the distance." He tells them not to focus on the middle of the journey, since that is often the most unpredictable part of the road to recovery. In short, Dr. Taylor suggests that you concentrate on what you need to do today to achieve your goals and then on how you will feel when you have completed the mending process. Dr. Taylor says, "Maintaining a long-term perspective is important. No one rehab session will predict your recovery."

For most people, healing takes more time than they'd like it to take, and the burden of the journey is lessened if they recognize and even celebrate their progress. Look back to where you started out and see how far you've come. If you achieve one of your goals, mark it with a celebration. This can be something simple such as buying yourself an inexpensive beaded bracelet as a visual reminder of the fact that you've accomplished your goal. Or, celebrate by doing something special that you've wanted to do—go to see a movie, eat at a favorite restaurant, or take a walk in the park. It really doesn't matter how you celebrate—just the act of commemorating your progress will help you during this journey.

Finally, above all else, keep in mind that people are extraordinarily resilient. We have many untapped resources that may have to be tapped during the healing process.

chapter 14

You Can Heal Yourself

One afternoon I had just settled into my seat on an airplane when there was a commotion a couple of rows behind me. Apparently, a young woman was taking a long time to get settled into her seat. She had her iPod on with earplugs and didn't realize the man standing behind her in the row was getting impatient. Other passengers saw his frustration and heard him make some disparaging remarks, however. Then, the commotion began. Finally fed up with this young woman, he decided to teach her a lesson and deliberately hit her with his carry-on bag—or so the witnesses reported. This man, a slightly overweight middle-aged businessman, vehemently denied that he struck her on purpose when the flight attendant told him the captain had insisted that he disembark. The man began arguing and demanded to talk to the captain personally. The plane was grounded as all of this took place and after about ten minutes, he came back to his seat, collected his belongings, and was escorted off the plane by the flight attendant. We then flew to our destination, minus one passenger.

Whether you are taking a real journey or a metaphorical healing journey, it takes time; rushing may lead to unintended and negative consequences. We'd all like to be at our desired destination instantaneously, but no journey works that way. The man on the plane needed to learn patience and respect. These qualities go a long way to helping people with their physical recovery as well: patience for the time it takes to heal, and respect for your body as it works to mend. I know this may be easier said than done, but consider the alternative. For the man on the plane, his journey no doubt took far longer to complete and perhaps with unanticipated obstacles to navigate as it was rumored on the plane that he went into the custody of airport security personnel. For the person who needs to heal, impatience can lead to setbacks, which can delay or even change the ultimate outcome.

There is no doubt that we are becoming increasingly accustomed to a very fast pace and nearly instant gratification. I remember when my son was in middle school and one day he texted me to pick him up after he finished band practice. Not more than fifteen minutes later I arrived, and he said, "Mom, what took you so long?" My son is a patient person by nature, but he was tired and hungry and had hours of homework in front of him. He was also firmly entrenched in the fast pace of the twenty-first century and waiting fifteen minutes seemed like a long time. All of my children and their friends, as well as most adults, have *expectations of speed*. However, these expectations don't usually work when it comes to healing. Instead, as my young saxophonist knew, musicians use the phrase *tempo giusto,* which means "the

right speed." In great music, as in healing, it is the right speed
that matters.

You Can Persevere

In a college course I took many years ago, a man named Dave
Scott was a guest speaker. What I remember most about his
talk was that he said he was never a stellar athlete. He rarely
took first place in any of the athletic events in which he com-
peted. However, he noticed that during practices, he was able
to last longer than anyone else. He had the most endurance
and he was able to persevere better than his teammates and
competitors. Scott decided to put his talent of perseverance
to use and began to compete in triathlons. His perseverance
led to astounding success and he became a six-time Ironman World Champion. (This triathlon takes place in Hawaii
and is a two-day event that includes a 2.4-mile swim, a 112-
mile bike ride, and a 26.2-mile marathon.) Not surprisingly,
Scott became the most recognized athlete in the sport of
triathlon and was the first inductee into the Ironman Hall of
Fame.

A dictionary definition of *persevere* is "to persist in a
state, enterprise, or undertaking in spite of counterinfluences,
opposition, or discouragement." Perseverance doesn't mean
that you are happy-go-lucky. Trying to heal is difficult, and
it's normal for people to feel discouraged at times. Helen Keller,
an icon of perseverance and success, once summed it up this
way: "I long to accomplish a great and noble task, but it is my

chief duty to accomplish small tasks as if they were great and noble." As you focus on healing, consider the "small accomplishments" that you make. These will add up, even if they don't seem like a big deal at the time.

After I was diagnosed with cancer, people were surprised, even my good friends, at how long it took me to really begin to feel like myself again. They wanted me to feel better right away, and though I wished for that, too, it just wasn't possible. I rarely discussed with others how much I was struggling during this time, but one day I was talking to my good friend and I was telling her how hard this journey really was. She was shocked and told me that she thought I was all better. She said, "But you walk around with a smile on your face. I had no idea you were still healing!" I realized then I had simply assumed those around me would know that I wasn't fully recovered and that my healing journey was taking many months. I also realized that by not specifically saying anything to my friend, she had mistakenly assumed that the fact that I was smiling and pleasant meant that I felt really good physically. I remember thinking to myself, "Wow, I faked out one of my closest friends!" But I didn't mean to. I just assumed some things and she assumed some things and neither of us really knew what the other was thinking.

This is a pretty common scenario—people tend to look better than they feel and if they don't specifically tell their loved ones what is going on, then those they are closest to assume they feel better than they do. Another way to think of this is that people tend to heal more quickly on the outside than they do on the inside. It simply takes longer for all of the different organs and tissues that we have inside our bodies to heal well. This occurred to me one day as a woman who is a cancer survivor and her best friend came up to me at a talk I was giving. She said, "My best friend knows that I still don't feel well, but my husband doesn't want to believe that I still don't feel well." I asked her a couple of questions about her husband and found out that he was generally a very kind and loving man. I suspect that two things may have created the misunderstanding between this couple. First, the wife may have assumed that her husband understood more than he did about how she was physically feeling. Just because her friend understands, doesn't mean that her husband might not need more explanation. Second, as often happens, those who love us most want so much for us to feel better that they may somewhat deceive themselves into believing it's true.

Since it took me approximately two years to heal optimally, the last thing I wanted to do was to confide in every person I met during that time about the fact that I was still mending. Instead, I learned to be honest and talk to the people closest to me in intervals. Obviously, incessant complaining doesn't help anyone, but it's a good idea to let your loved ones know how you feel; it's helpful to do this once in a while so that they—and you—don't feel the constant burden of the healing journey.

Of course, when I say that I felt about 90 percent better after two years, I am just estimating. But, it took me about that long to be close to feeling as good as I was going to ever feel again—which wasn't quite as good as I would have felt if I had never had cancer or cancer treatment, but it was still much, much better than I felt at the end of my chemotherapy regimen. I say 90 percent, because almost everyone who has endured serious health issues, including me, has areas that they can continue to work on.

For me to write that I was patient throughout my recovery would not be accurate. Unlike my son, I'm not naturally inclined to be patient. However, one thing that helped me relax and accept what often seemed to be the very slow pace of physical healing was the knowledge that I was doing what I could to provide my body with what it needed to facilitate recovery. Basically I was doing everything I could to heal. This doesn't mean that I did everything exactly right; it wouldn't be true and would be practically impossible to do over the course of a year or more. There were days that I ate too much junk food and days when I moped instead of going out to exercise. There were many nights, especially in the beginning, when no matter what I did, I couldn't sleep a solid eight hours. Yet, I recovered as well as possible because what it really means to heal optimally is to:

- focus on the strategies that you think will help you;
- consider your goals;
- expect some setbacks and don't let them derail your journey either physically or emotionally;
- do the best you can—keeping in mind that your body wants to heal, and any help you give it is extremely valuable.

Healing as Well as Possible

There are tremendous and often unforeseen benefits of using healing strategies. They can create new habits that can last a lifetime and be extremely beneficial to you as you age. The good news is that after you heal optimally, you don't have to do any extra work to create these great health habits—you just need to keep doing what you've been doing all along.

I often tell the story of my mother-in-law who was struck down by a stroke when she was in her early forties. With eight children to raise, she worked extremely hard to heal. Though her recovery took time, she focused on the most important aspects of healing and these became lifetime habits. Today she is in her seventies and she is quite remarkable in her vigor and good health. There is no doubt that her stroke propelled her to make some lifestyle changes that facilitated not only her stroke recovery but also had dramatic effects on her health throughout her life.

Some people might see this as a "gift" that comes out of a serious illness. I have a hard time seeing any illness as a gift, but I do think that every experience, whether it's good or bad, provides us with opportunities for change. Facing serious illness allows one to stop and reflect in a way that might not otherwise be possible. Out of this can come some wonderful opportunities to choose a new direction or path that one might not have previously considered taking.

I have seen thousands of people heal optimally, and no journey was exactly the same as any other. Most of the people

I shepherd through their recovery, whether they have a new injury or illness or a chronic one, come to accept whatever limitations they have to. This doesn't mean they are happy about these limitations; it just means they are able to move beyond them and lead meaningful lives.

While most individuals strike a balance between working hard to recover and accepting whatever losses they must endure, there are two groups of people who end up with more disability than they need to live with. The first group consists of those who are overly accepting of their limitations. These folks just assume that as we age, we become very decrepit and so it's better to just go along with this rather than to fight it. This attitude is not based in science, which shows that as we age, we can make tremendous gains in our physical endurance, strength, mobility, and so on, by employing much of what I have outlined in this book. The second group who don't heal as well as they can consists of people who are unwilling to accept any limitations. They want to be just as they were "before" and if this isn't possible, they simply give up trying to mend.

Healing optimally is often about compromise. You have to settle for less than you want in order to have the best outcome. These are lessons that we have had to learn throughout our lives, though a few people will always opt out if they can't get exactly what they want. This path reminds me of a story my daughter told me many years ago about her schoolyard playmates. There was one strong-willed child who wanted to control all of the games. This little girl was the self-appointed leader and would select my daughter and another child to play with. Then, when a fourth girl asked to play, the leader would promptly tell her, "This game can only be played with three kids." My daughter didn't like this, so she told the fourth child, "Of course you can play, and we'll take turns or make teams." Whereupon the leader, desperately trying to maintain control responded with, "Okay, then I'm not going to play."

These were innocent children who had much to learn about compromise, leadership, and friendship, and the playground is a place where they practiced these skills. In healing, compromise is a part of the process. Employing the child-leader's technique of opting out when she doesn't get exactly what she wants is not ideal on the playground. Nor is it useful when trying to recover optimally.

Once you commit yourself to a given task, things often fall into place in a manner that you couldn't have predicted. It is as if the stars align and work with you. In a passage from *The Scottish Himalayan Expedition,* W. H. Murray explains how commitment works:

> Until one is committed, there is hesitancy. . . . The moment one definitely commits oneself, then Providence moves, too. All sorts of things occur to help one that would never otherwise have occurred. A whole stream of events raising in one's favor . . . unforeseen incidents and meetings and material assistance which no man could have dreamed could have come his way.

I encourage you to commit yourself to healing as well as you can. Make your journey as safe a passage as possible. Work hard and diligently to insure that your final destination is the best place you can arrive at. Know that there will be bumps in the road—accept them, change your navigation as needed, and continue your journey.

One of my patients had a back operation and asked me what he could do for me since I had helped him with his rehabilitation. My first instinct was to say "nothing" but then I decided that I really did want something. I wanted to know that now that he felt better, he would pursue the travel he had been longing to do. So I said, "Every time you go somewhere, send me a magnet with the name of the city you are in." This amazing man filled my refrigerator with magnets, and my kids would marvel at all of the exotic places he traveled to.

Humorist Doc Blakey once said, "Success is getting up just one more time than you fall down." Both Abraham Lincoln and Winston Churchill are notorious for their many, many failures before achieving success. Churchill had a lifetime of adversity before he finally became the prime minister of England when he was sixty-two years of age—then considered a "senior citizen." As a world leader, he personified the attitude of perseverance and rallied the spirits and the action of a nation when they were against the superior German forces in World War II. In his later years, Churchill was invited to address students at Harrow School. Churchill's advice to the students is the same as my final words to end this book: "Never, never, never give up."

appendix

Where to Find Help

Medical Information

American Academy of Physical Medicine and Rehabilitation
(AAPM&R)
9700 West Bryn Mawr Avenue, Suite 200
Rosemont, IL 60018-5701
847-737-6000
www.aapmr.org

The AAPM&R is the premier national medical society for physicians who specialize in physical medicine and rehabilitation. The
Web site has sections for membership, the annual assembly, physicians, residents, medical students, and continuing medical education. There is also industry information and a job board.

American Cancer Society (ACS)
2970 Clairmont Road NE
Atlanta, GA 30329-1638
800-ACS-2345 (800-227-2345)
www.cancer.org

The ACS is a nationwide community-based volunteer health organization with state divisions and more than 3,400 local offices.

The goal of the ACS is to eliminate cancer as a major health problem by preventing the disease, saving lives, and diminishing suffering through research, education, advocacy, and service. The Web site has sections for patients, families and friends, survivors, donors and volunteers, and professionals.

American Medical Association (AMA)
515 N State Street
Chicago, IL 60654-9104
800-621-8335 or 312-464-5000
www.ama-assn.org

The AMA, the country's largest physician's group, develops and promotes standards in medical practice, research, and education. The consumer health information section on the association's Web site has databases on physicians and hospitals that can be searched by medical specialty, as well as information on specific conditions.

National Center for Complementary and Alternative
    Medicine (NCCAM)
P.O. Box 7923
Gaithersburg, MD 20898
1-888-466-6226 or 866-464-3613 (TYY) or 301-231-7537,
    ext. 5 (from outside the U.S.)
www.nccam.nih.gov

NCCAM explores complementary and alternative healing practices through research, research training and education, outreach, and integration. The NCCAM Web site offers publications, information for researchers, frequently asked questions, and links to other CAM-related resources. The NCCAM Clearinghouse is the public's source for scientifically based information on CAM and for information about NCCAM.

National Institutes of Health (NIH)
9000 Rockville Pike

Bethesda, MD 20892
301-496-4000 or 301-402-9612 (TTY)
http://nih.gov

The NIH is a focal point for medical research in the United States, and is comprised of 27 institutes and centers. It is an agency of the Public Health Service, which is a division of the U.S. Department of Health and Human Services. NIH research acquires new knowledge to help prevent, detect, diagnose, and treat disease and disability.

National Library of Medicine (NLM)
8600 Rockville Pike
Bethesda, MD 20894
888-FINDNLM (888-346-3656)
www.nlm.nih.gov

The NLM collects, organizes, and makes available biomedicine and health care information to medical professionals and offers programs for medical library services in the United States. Both health professionals and the public use its electronic databases extensively throughout the world. Materials are available in multiple languages.

Susan G. Komen Breast Cancer Foundation
5005 LBJ Freeway, Suite 250
Dallas, TX 75244
1-877-GO-KOMAN (1-877-465-6636)
http://ww5.komen.org

The Susan G. Komen Breast Cancer Foundation is a global leader in the fight against breast cancer. It funds research grants and supports education, screening, and treatment projects in communities around the world. In addition to information about breast cancer, the Web site contains information about obtaining grants, making donations, participating in events, subscribing to free newsletters, and purchasing gifts and educational materials from the Foundation.

Nutrition

American Dietetic Association (ADA)
120 South Riverside Plaza, Suite 2000
Chicago, IL 60606-6995
800-877-1600 or 312-899-0040
www.eatright.org

The ADA, the world's largest organization of food and nutrition professionals, promotes nutrition, health, and well-being. The Web site has information on diet and nutrition and publications, as well as a registered dietitian locator service, which includes dietitians who specialize in oncology nutrition.

Harvard School of Public Health
Department of Nutrition
665 Huntington Avenue
Boston, MA 02115
617-432-1851
www.hsph.harvard.edu/nutritionsource

The Nutrition Source is a Web site that is maintained by the Department of Nutrition at the Harvard School of Public Health. The Web site serves as a resource for the most up-to-date information on diet and nutrition and dispels rumors and fallacies about fad diets.

International Food Information Council (IFIC) Foundation
1100 Connecticut Avenue NW, Suite 430
Washington, D.C. 20036
202-296-6540
www.foodinsight.org/

The IFIC Foundation offers science-based information on food safety and nutrition to health and nutrition professionals, educators, journalists, and others. The IFIC partners with a wide range of professional organizations and academic institutions to develop science-based information for the public.

Meals-on-Wheels Association of America (MOWAA)
203 S. Union Street
Alexandria, VA 22314
703-548-5558
www.mowaa.org

Meals-on-Wheels is a membership association that offers programs to provide home-delivered and group meals. The organization aims to improve the quality of life of the needy. Some programs may provide other health and social services.

National Heart, Lung, and Blood Institute Health
    Information Center
P.O. Box 30105
Bethesda, MD 20824-0104
301-592-8573
http://nhlbisupport.com/bmi

This Web site provides information about body mass index and what constitutes a healthy weight for both men and women. The Web site also provides links to information about controlling food and planning menus.

The Office of Dietary Supplements (ODS)
National Institutes of Health
6100 Executive Blvd., Room 3B01, MSC 7517
Bethesda, MD 20892-7517
301-435-2920
http://ods.od.nih.gov

The ODS supports research and publishes results about dietary supplements. It plans, organizes, and supports scientific conferences, workshops, and symposia on topics related to dietary supplements.

USDA Food and Nutrition Information Center (FNIC)
National Agricultural Library
10301 Baltimore Avenue, Room 105
Beltsville, MD 20705-2351
301-504-5414
http://nal.usda.gov/fnic

The USDA's FNIC is an information center for the National Agricultural Library. FNIC materials and services include dietitians
and nutritionists available to answer inquiries, publications on
food and nutrition, and resource lists and bibliographies. The
FNIC Web site includes information on dietary supplements,
food safety, dietary guidelines, food composition facts (including
fast food), a list of available publications, and information on
popular topics.

United States Food and Drug Administration (FDA)
5600 Fishers Lane
Rockville, MD 20857-0001
888-INFO-FDA (888-463-6332)
www.fda.gov

The FDA is a public health agency that enforces the Federal Food,
Drug, and Cosmetic Act among other laws, promotes health by
helping safe and effective products reach the market in a timely
manner, and monitors products for continued safety once they are
in use. The Web site has information on FDA-regulated products.

Pain

American Academy of Pain Medicine (AAPM)
4700 West Lake Avenue
Glenview, IL 60025
847-375-4731
www.painmed.org

The AAPM is the medical specialty society for physicians practic-
ing pain medicine. The AAPM is involved in education, training,

advocacy, and research in pain medicine. The Web site has links to other sites related to pain and pain medicine. The Web site also features membership information and links to the Academy's publications and products.

American Chronic Pain Association (ACPA)
P.O. Box 850
Rocklin, CA 95677-0850
800-533-3231
www.theacpa.org
e-mail: acpa@pacbell.net

The ACPA offers information and support for people with chronic pain and their families. The ACPA also strives to raise awareness among those in the medical profession, policy makers, and the general public about living with chronic pain. The Web site has some free, downloadable information about managing pain, as well as an online store where videos, manuals, and other materials can be purchased.

American Pain Foundation
201 N. Charles Street, Suite 710
Baltimore, MD 21201-4111
888-615-PAIN (888-615-7246)
http://painfoundation.org

This independent nonprofit organization provides information, education, and advocacy to people with pain. The foundation's Web site has a pain information library, downloadable publications, and useful links about pain.

American Pain Society
4700 West Lake Avenue
Glenview, IL 60025
847-375-4715
www.ampainsoc.org
e-mail: info@ampainsoc.org

The American Pain Society, a nonprofit membership organization of scientists, clinicians, policy analysts, and others, seeks to advance pain-related research, education, treatment, and professional practice. The Web site provides limited publications on pain, which can either be viewed online or ordered for a fee.

Mental Health

American Association for Marriage and Family Therapy
    (AAMFT)
112 South Alfred Street
Alexandria, VA 22314-3061
703-838-9808 or 202-452-0109
www.aamft.org

The AAMFT is the professional organization for marriage and family therapists. In addition to resources for professionals, the organization provides the public with referrals to marriage and family therapists. It also provides educational materials on living with illness and other issues related to families and health.

American Counseling Association (ACA)
5999 Stevenson Avenue
Alexandria, VA 22304-3300
800-347-6647
http://counseling.org

The ACA is a nonprofit professional and educational organization that supports the counseling profession. The Web site has information for students, consumers, and counselors.

American Psychiatric Association (APA)
1000 Wilson Boulevard, Suite 1825
Arlington, VA 22209-3901
1-888-35-PSYCH (1-888-357-7924)
www.psych.org

The APA is a medical specialty society. The 35,000+ U.S. and international physicians belonging to the APA work together to provide humane care and effective treatment for anyone with mental disorders, including mental retardation and substance-related disorders. The Web site includes information about the APA and links to related organizations.

American Psychological Association (APA)
750 First Street NE
Washington, D.C. 2002-4242
800-374-2721 or 202-336-6123 (TDD/TTY)
http://apa.org

The APA offers referrals to psychologists in local areas and provides information on family issues, parenting, and health. The APA Web site has links to state psychological associations that may also provide local referrals.

National Association of Social Workers (NASW)
750 First Street, NE, Suite 700
Washington, D.C. 20002-4241
202-408-8600
www.socialworkers.org

The NASW is the world's largest membership organization of professional social workers. The NASW enhances the professional growth and development of its members, creates and maintains professional standards, and advances sound social policies. The Web site has information and links for professionals and the general public. The NASW's publications can be ordered online for a fee.

Spiritual

American Association of Pastoral Counselors
9504A Lee Highway
Fairfax, VA 22031-2302

703-385-6967
http://aapc.org

The American Association of Pastoral Counselors offers an online directory of Certified Pastoral Counselors across the country, as well as links to other relevant resources.

Caregivers and Other Support

Air Charity Network
4620 Haygood Road, Suite 1
Viriginia Beach, VA 23455
800-549-9980 or 877-621-7177

This nonprofit organization provides free flights by volunteer pilots, who use their own private planes to transport patients who cannot afford the cost of commercial flights to their medical facility.

American Association of Retired People (AARP)
601 E Street, NW
Washington D.C. 20049
888-OUR-AARP (888-687-2277)
www.aarp.org
aarppharmacy.com (Pharmacy Service)

AARP is a nonprofit membership organization open to anyone fifty years old and older. Its member services include information on managed and long-term care, Medicare, and Medicaid. The Web site has information on a pharmacy service that offers discounts on drugs used for cancer treatment and pain relief.

National Family Caregivers Association (NFCA)
10400 Connecticut Avenue, Suite 500
Kensington, MD 20895-3944
1-800-896-3650
www.nfcacares.org
e-mail: info@nfcacares.org

The NFCA provides education, support, and advocacy for family caregivers. The Web site offers publications and other materials for purchase, as well as some free, downloadable information. There are also links to other Web sites that provide information about specific diseases and disabilities, as well as other health-care issues.

The Well Spouse Foundation
63 West Main Street, Suite H
Freehold, NJ 07728
800-838-0879
www.wellspouse.org
e-mail: info@wellspouse.org

Well Spouse is a national, not-for-profit membership organization that offers support to wives, husbands, and partners of the chronically ill and/or disabled. Well Spouse support groups meet monthly. The Web site provides information about how to become a member, meeting times and places, activities, conferences, printed material, and links to other relevant organizations.

Other

American Association of Sex Educators, Counselors, and
    Therapists (AASECT)
1444 I Street, NW, Suite 700
Washington, D.C. 20005
202-449-1099
http://aasect.org

The AASECT is a nonprofit, interdisciplinary professional organization that promotes understanding human sexuality and healthy sexual behavior. In addition to sex educators, sex counselors, and sex therapists, AASECT members include physicians, nurses, social workers, psychologists, allied health professionals, clergy members, lawyers, sociologists, marriage and family planning specialists, and researchers, as well as students in relevant professional disciplines. The Web site offers information for the public and professionals, with links to a variety of related organizations.

Council of State Administrators of Vocational Rehabilitation
    (CSAVR)
1 Research Court, Suite 450
Rockville, MD 20850
301-519-8023
www.rehabnetwork.org

The CSAVR consists of the chief administrators of the public rehabilitation agencies, which serve individuals with physical and mental disabilities in the United States and its territories. The CSAVR is the only national organization that advocates for the Public Vocational Rehabilitation Program. The mission is to maintain and enhance a national program of public vocational rehabilitation services so that individuals with disabilities can achieve employment, economic self-sufficiency, independence, and inclusion and integration into the community.

references

Chapter 1

Michael, Jan. *Flying Crooked*. Vancouver, BC: Greystone Books, 2005.

Silver, Julie. *After Cancer Treatment: Heal Faster, Better, Stronger.* Baltimore, MD: Johns Hopkins University Press, 2006.

Sontag, Susan. *Illness as Metaphor and AIDS and Its Metaphors*. New York: Picador, 2001.

Chapter 2

Frankl, Viktor. *Man's Search for Meaning*. Boston: Beacon Press, 2006.

Osborn, Claudia L. *Over My Head*. Kansas City, MO: Andrews McMeel Publishing, 1998.

Chapter 3

Bennett, Arnold. *How to Live on 24 Hours a Day*. Hyattsville, MD: Shambling Gates Press, 2000.

Woolf, Virginia. "On Being Ill." In *The Moment and Other Essays*. New York: Harcourt Brace & Company, 1974.

Chapter 4

Benson, Herbert. *The Relaxation Response*. New York: HarperCollins, 2000.

Cousins, Norman. *Anatomy of an Illness as Perceived by the Patient*. New York, W. W. Norton, 1979.

Dreher, Henry. *Mind-Body Unity*. Baltimore: The Johns Hopkins University Press, 2003.

Chapter 5

Domar, Alice, and Henry Dreher. *Self-Nurture*. New York: Penguin, 2000.

Heller, Richard and Rachael Heller. *Healthy Selfishness*. Des Moines, IA: Meredith Books, 2006.

Ornish, Dean. *Love and Survival*. New York: Harper Collins, 1998.

Chapter 6

Frank, Arthur W. *At the Will of the Body*. Boston: Mariner Books, 2002.

Holland, Jimmie C., and Sheldon Lewis. *The Human Side of Cancer*. New York: Quill, 2000.

Laurent, C. "Wounds heal more quickly if patients are relieved of stress." In *British Medical Journal* 327 (2003): 522.

Marucha, P. T. et al. "Mucosal wound healing is impaired by examination stress." In *Psychosomatic Medicine* 60 (1998): 362–65.

Meili, Trisha. *I Am the Central Park Jogger*. New York: Scribner, 2003.

Silver, Julie. *After Cancer Treatment*. Baltimore: The Johns Hopkins University Press, 2006.

Westberg, Granger E. *Good Grief*. Minneapolis: Fortress Press, 1997.

Chapter 7

Carroll, L. J., J. D. Cassidy, and P. Cote. "Frequency, timing and course for depressive symptomatology after whiplash." In *Spine* 31 (2006): E551–56.

Cremeans-Smith, J. K., K. Millington, E. Sledjeski, K. Greene, and D. K. Delahanty. "Sleep disruptions mediate the relationship between early postoperative pain and later functioning following total knee replacement surgery." In Journal of Behavioral Medicine 2 (2006): 215–222.

Chapter 8

Coyne J. C., M. J. Rohrbaugh, V. Shoham, J. S. Sonnega, J. M. Nicklas, and J. A. Cranford. "Prognostic importance of marital quality for survival of congestive heart failure." In *American Journal of Cardiology* 88 (2001): 526–9.

Eaker, E. D., L. M. Sullivan, M. Kelly-Hayes, R.B. D'Agostino Sr., and E. J. Benjamin. "Marital status, marital strain, and risk of coronary heart disease or total mortality: the Framingham Offspring Study." In *Psychosomatic Medicine* 69(6) (2007): 509–13.

Glynn, L.M., N. Christenfeld, and W. Gerin. "Gender, social support, and cardiovascular responses to stress." In *Psychosomatic Medicine* 1999; 61: 234–42.

Gore, J. L., L. Kwan, C. S. Saigal, and M.S. Litwin. "Marriage and mortality in bladder carcinoma." In *Cancer* 2005;104:1188–94.

Hallowell, Edward M. *Connect*. New York: Pocket Books, 1999.

Kiecolt-Glaser, J. K., et al. "Hostile Marital interactions, proinflammatory cytokine production, and wound healing." In *Archives of General Psychiatry* 62 (2005): 1377–84.

Kiecolt-Glaser, J. K., et al. "Negative Behavior During Marital Conflict is Associated with Immunological Down-Regulation." In *Psychosomatic Medicine* 55.5 (1993): 395–409.

Kraut, R. et al. "Internet paradox: a social technology that reduces social involvement and psychological well-being?" In *The American Psychologist* 53 (1998): 1017–31.

Lerner, Harriet. *The Dance of Connection*. New York: Quill, 2002.

Lucas, Geralyn. *Why I Wore Lipstick to My Mastectomy*. New York: St. Martin's Griffin, 2004.

Muizzuddin, N., M. S. Matsui, K. D. Marenus, and D.H. Maes. "Impact of stress of marital dissolution on skin barrier recovery: tape stripping and measurement of trans-epidermal water loss (TEWL)." In *Skin Research and Technology* (2003): 9:34–8.

Orth-Gomér, K., S. P. Wamala, M. Horsten, K. Schenck-Gustafsson, N. Schneiderman, and M. A. Mittleman. "Marital stress worsens prognosis in women with coronary heart disease: The Stockholm Female Coronary Risk Study." In *Journal of the American Medical Association* 284 (2000): 3008–14.

Rodgers, Joni. *Bald in the Land of Big Hair.* New York: HarperCollins, 2001.

Saper, R. B. et al. "Heavy Metal content of ayurvedic herbal medicine products." In *Journal of the American Medical Association* 292 (2004): 2868–73.

Chapter 9

Crews, F. T. et al. "Cytokines and Alcohol." In *Alcoholism: Clinical and Experimental Research* 30 (2006): 720–30.

Degoutte, F. et al. "Food restriction, performance, biochemical, psychological, and endocrine changes in judo athletes." In *International Journal of Sports Medicine* 27 (2006): 9–18.

Frieman, A. et al. "Cutaneous effects of smoking." In *Journal of Cutaneous Medicine and Surgery* 8 (2004): 415–23.

Saper, R. B. et al. "Heavy Metal content of ayurvedic herbal medicine products." In *Journal of the American Medical Association* 292 (2004): 2868–73.

Chapter 10

Csikszentmihalyi, Mihaly. *Flow: The Psychology of Optimal Experience.* New York: Harper Perennial, 1990.

Emery, C. F. et al. "Exercise Accelerates wound healing among healthy older adults: A preliminary investigation." In *Journal of Gerontology* 11 (2005): 1432–36.

Chapter 11

Epstein, Lawrence, and Steve Mardon. *The Harvard Medical School Guide to a Good Night's Sleep.* New York: McGraw-Hill, 2006.

Jones, C. B. et al. "Fatigue and the criminal law." In *Industrial Health* 43 (2005) 63–70.

Malik, S. W., and J. Kaplan. "Sleep deprivation." In *Primary Care: Clinics in Office Practice* 32 (2005): 475–90.

Parthasarathy, S., and M. J. Tobin. "Sleep in the intensive care unit." In *Intensive Care Medicine* 30 (2004): 197–206.

Rogers, N. L. et al. "Neuroimmunologic aspects of sleep and sleep loss." In *Seminars in Clinical Neuropsychiatry* 6 (2001): 295–307.

Chapter 12

Boudreaux, E. D. et al. "Spiritual role in healing: An alternative way of thinking." In *Primary Care* 29 (2002): 439–54.

Karff, Samuel E. "Healing of boy, healing of spirit." In *CCAR Journal: A Reform Jewish Quarterly* (2004): 85–95.

Kliewer, S. "Allowing spirituality into the healing process." In *The Journal of Family Practice* 53 (2004): 616–24.

Kushner, Harold. *Who Needs God.* New York: Fireside, 1989.

MacNutt, Francis. *The Power to Heal.* Notre Dame, IN: Ave Maria Press, 2004.

Marty, Martin E. "Religion and Healing: The Four Expectations." In *Religion and Healing in America,* edited by Linda L. Barns and Susan S. Sered. New York: Oxford University Press, 2005.

Phillips, Robert H. *Rising to the Challenge: Celebrities and Their Very Personal Health Stories.* Garden City Park, NY: Avery Publishing Group, 1990.

Shuman, Joel James, and Keith G. Meador. *Heal Thyself: Spirituality, Medicine, and the Distortion of Christianity.* New York: Oxford University Press, 2003.

Silver, Julie K., M.D. *What Helped Get Me Through: Cancer Survivors Share Wisdom and Hope.* Atlanta, GA: American Cancer Society, 2009.

Chapter 14

Murray, W. H. *The Scottish Himalayan Expedition.* London: J. M. Dent & Sons, 1951.

index